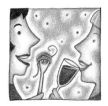

HEALTH AND HEALING
THE NATURAL WAY

———

ENERGISE
YOUR LIFE

———

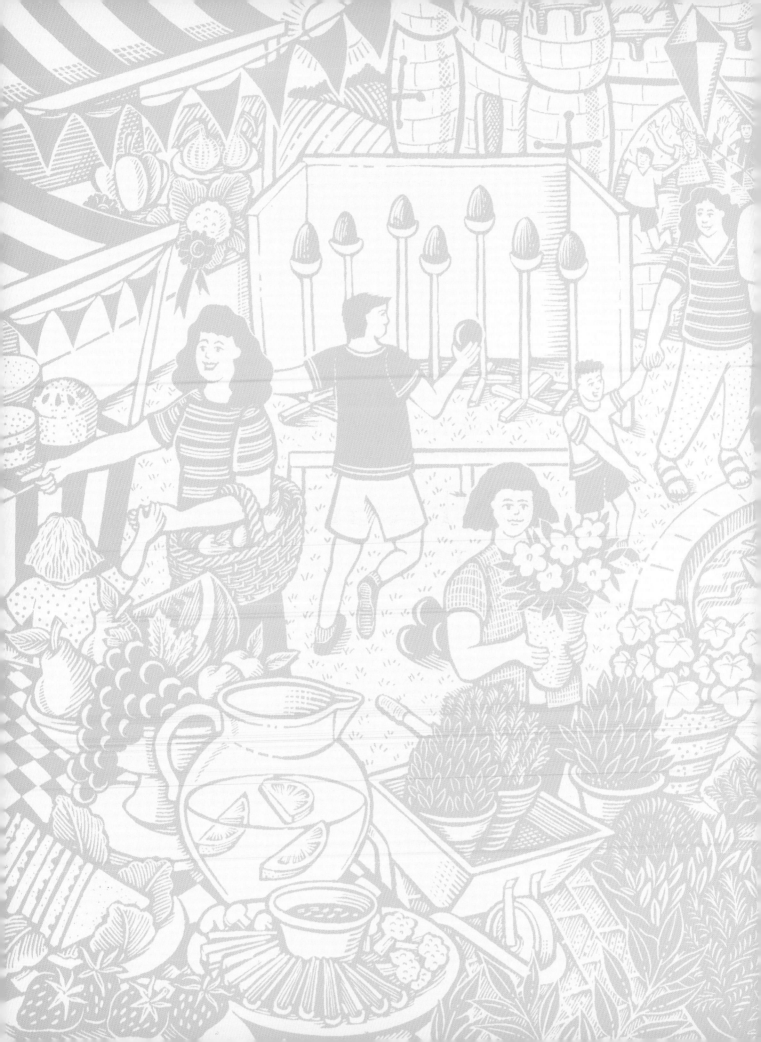

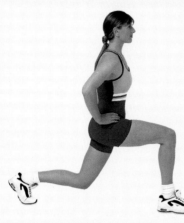

HEALTH AND HEALING THE NATURAL WAY

ENERGISE YOUR LIFE

Reader's
Digest

PUBLISHED BY

THE READER'S DIGEST ASSOCIATION LIMITED

LONDON NEW YORK SYDNEY MONTREAL CAPE TOWN

ENERGISE YOUR LIFE
was created and produced by
Carroll & Brown Limited
20 Lonsdale Road, London NW6 6RD
for The Reader's Digest Association Limited, London

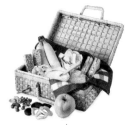

CARROLL & BROWN

Publishing Director Denis Kennedy
Art Director Chrissie Lloyd

Managing Editor Sandra Rigby
Managing Art Editor Tracy Timson

Editor Jennifer Mussett

Art Editors Mercedes Pearson, Sandra Brooke
Designers Vimit Punater, Julie Bennett

Photographers Jules Selmes, David Murray

Production Wendy Rogers, Clair Reynolds

Computer Management John Clifford,
Paul Stradling, Elisa Merino

First English Edition Copyright © 1999
The Reader's Digest Association Limited,
11 Westferry Circus, Canary Wharf,
London E14 4HE

Copyright © 1999
The Reader's Digest Association Far East Limited
Philippines Copyright © 1999
The Reader's Digest Association Far East Limited

ISBN 0 276 42274 0

Reproduced by Colourscan, Singapore
Printing and binding: Printer Industria Gráfica S.A., Barcelona

CONSULTANT

Dr Michael Jenkins
MBBS, MRCP, FFHom
General practitioner and complementary health specialist

MEDICAL ILLUSTRATIONS CONSULTANT

Dr Amanda Roberts
MA, MB, BChir

CONTRIBUTORS

Professor Peter O. Behan
MB, ChB, MD, DSc, FRCP (Glas),
FRCP (Lond), FRCP (I)
Professor of Neurology

Dr Abhijit Chaudhuri
DM, MD, MB, BSc, MRCP (UK)
University lecturer in neurology

Sue Thurgood
BSc, SRD
Senior dietitian

Richard Emerson
Medical health writer

Roger Newman Turner
BAc, ND, DO, MRO, MRN
Registered naturopath, osteopath and acupuncturist

FOR THE READER'S DIGEST

Series Editor Christine Noble
Editorial Assistant Caroline Boucher

READER'S DIGEST GENERAL BOOKS

Editorial Director Cortina Butler
Art Director Nick Clark

The information in this book is for reference only;
it is not intended as a substitute for a doctor's diagnosis and care.
The editors urge anyone with continuing medical problems
or symptoms to consult a doctor.

ENERGISE YOUR LIFE

More and more people today are choosing to take greater responsibility for their own health rather than relying on the doctor to step in with a cure when something goes wrong. We now recognise that we can influence our health by making an improvement in lifestyle – a better diet, more exercise and reduced stress. People are also becoming increasingly aware that there are other healing methods – some new, others very ancient – that can help to prevent illness or be used as a complement to orthodox medicine.

The series *Health and Healing the Natural Way* will help you to make your own health choices by giving you clear, comprehensive, straightforward and encouraging information and advice about methods of improving your health. The series explains the many different natural therapies now available – aromatherapy, herbalism, acupressure and many others – and the circumstances in which they may be of benefit when used in conjunction with conventional medicine.

ENERGISE YOUR LIFE investigates the causes of and treatments for fatigue and energy problems, and provides energy-boosting suggestions for cases ranging from those who feel tired at times to those with a major debilitating condition. All of the main causes of fatigue are covered, including sleeping problems, emotional stress, lifestyle and illness. There is an in-depth analysis of dietary needs and the use of nutrient supplements in the treatment of energy problems. The book also describes energising exercises for your body and your mind, and how you can reduce stress and other energy drainers in your lifestyle. Finally, the book covers the main medical conditions that can lead to fatigue and some of the complementary therapies that can help to alleviate them. *ENERGISE YOUR LIFE* shows how we can all develop and maintain a more positive outlook to promote inproved health and vitality and a sense of balance in life.

CONTENTS

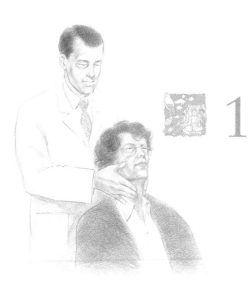

INTRODUCTION: BOOSTING ENERGY LEVELS 8

 1 ENERGY AND THE INDIVIDUAL

WHAT IS ENERGY? 16

ENERGY AND YOUR BODY 18

The endocrinologist 26

WOMEN AND ENERGY 29

Combating tiredness during pregnancy 32

The fatigued solicitor 35

MEN AND ENERGY 36

Self-help to counter impotence 37

2 THE ENERGY ALL AROUND US

LIGHT AND COLOUR 40

Improving your mood with colour therapy 41

The power of magnetism 43

SOUND 44

Expressing your emotions with sound therapy 45

ANIMALS, VEGETABLES AND MINERALS 46

THE FIVE ENERGIES 48

Ayurveda practitioner 50

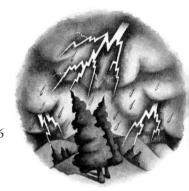

 3 ENERGY DRAINERS

SLEEP AND ENERGY 54

Dealing with snoring 58

EMOTIONAL DRAIN ON ENERGY 60

The perfectionist 61

Preventing and coping with burnout 63

ALLERGIES AND INTOLERANCES 64

ENVIRONMENTAL FACTORS 66

CHRONIC PAIN 68

Relieving chronic pain fatigue with natural pain beaters 70

DIETS THAT DRAIN ENERGY 72

The caffeine addict 73

Methods to counter daytime drowsiness 76

DRUGS THAT DRAIN ENERGY 78

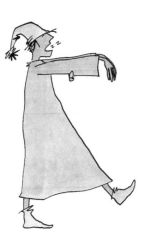

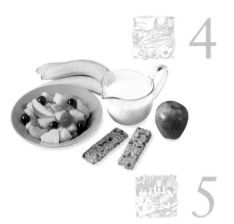

4 EATING FOR ENERGY

THE COMPONENTS OF HEALTHY EATING *82*

A constantly tired woman *87*

ENERGY LEVELS THROUGH THE DAY *88*

ENERGY LEVELS AND SPECIAL DIETS *90*

Retaining high energy levels while losing weight *93*

THE ENERGY NUTRIENTS *94*

5 A VITAL MIND AND BODY

REGULAR EXERCISE FOR ENERGY *112*

Boosting energy with a home work-out *114*

ENERGY AND YOUR EMOTIONS *119*

The chi kung teacher *120*

Clear your mind with standing meditation *123*

The irritable mother *125*

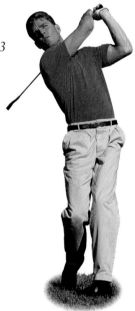

6 SERIOUS CONDITIONS AND ILLNESSES

CONSULTING YOUR DOCTOR *128*

HIGH OR LOW BLOOD PRESSURE *130*

HEART AND ARTERY DISEASE *132*

LUNG DISORDERS *134*

ANAEMIA *136*

ADRENAL GLAND PROBLEMS *138*

THYROID PROBLEMS *140*

DIABETES *142*

HYPOGLYCAEMIA *144*

CANCER *146*

HIV AND AIDS *148*

ME (CHRONIC FATIGUE SYNDROME) *150*

VIRAL INFECTIONS *154*

INDEX *157*

ACKNOWLEDGMENTS *160*

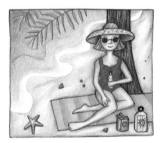

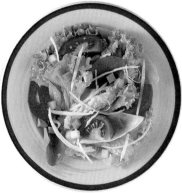

BOOSTING ENERGY LEVELS

Most people would like more energy to cope with life's demands and, in many cases, simple lifestyle changes can give rich rewards in energy levels.

In recent years lack of energy has become a major health issue. It is one of the most common complaints presented to doctors and is the subject of hundreds of magazine articles, TV chat shows and self-help books. People often complain that if only they had more energy they could achieve more, be happier, or even simply stay on top of existing commitments. Although we all suffer periods of low energy from time to time, for some people loss of energy takes an extreme and disabling form: chronic fatigue syndrome.

Chronic fatigue syndrome or CFS (also known as ME) remains a controversial condition in the eyes of some medical practitioners. Increasingly, however, doctors are recognising it as a distinct and diagnosable illness. It is now generally defined as extreme fatigue; in some cases the sufferer is unable even to move without assistance. Exactly what causes CFS is unclear, although it often appears to follow a severe flu-like virus. A number of risk factors have been identified: protracted physical or mental stress, nutritional deficiencies and allergies can all unbalance the immune system and appear to make some people vulnerable to extreme fatigue. The condition seems to be on the increase; it is conservatively estimated to affect 40 people per 100 000, although US studies suggest the figure could be as high as 100 per 100 000.

There are many theories as to why fatigue is on the increase in the late 20th century. Some people believe our modern lifestyle is simply too demanding; that the pace of life causes excessive mental and physical stress which depletes the immune system. Other people believe that low energy reflects a depressed outlook, or bad eating habits, or too little or even too much exercise. The reality seems to be that low energy is the result of a complex interaction of all of these factors, and treatments need to encompass the whole being. However, not only are the causes of low energy diverse; the concept of what we actually mean by energy has also broadened in recent

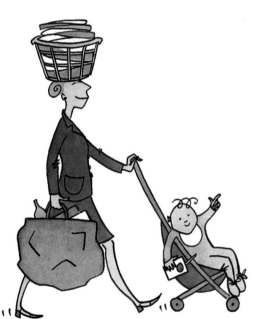

BUSY, BUSY WORLD
More is expected of everyone in today's fast-moving world. Getting everything done and staying on top of commitments can demand high levels of energy.

years. What scientists have learnt has had huge implications not only for the way we look at the world around us, but also for how we understand our own health and energy levels.

SIR ISAAC NEWTON AND ENERGY

Up until the mid 19th century, our understanding of what energy consisted of, and how the physical world worked, even how the human body worked, was reasonably straightforward. The prevailing view of the world was largely based on the work of Sir Isaac Newton. He determined that the world consisted of solid units of matter (atoms) which always remained identical in shape and mass, and which were acted on by the force of gravity, which he saw as the essential energy force in the world. He believed that the world ran according to fixed rules like a giant machine, and that for every observable effect there was an identifiable cause. However, this theory failed to explain powerful energy forces discovered in the 19th century – electric and magnetic phenomena. By the mid 19th century, scientists had realised that the physical world and our own place in it was more complex than they had previously thought.

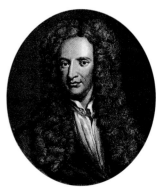

SIR ISAAC NEWTON
One of the greatest scientists in history, Newton believed that everything in the Universe was made from solid particles of matter, or atoms.

THE NEW PHYSICS

A radical shift in how science viewed the physical world occurred at the beginning of the 20th century when Albert Einstein published his theory of relativity and quantum theory. Until Einstein's discoveries, scientists from ancient Greek times onwards believed that all matter was composed of hard and solid particles. Einstein's theories, and the work of the physicists who followed him, showed that far from being solid, atoms consist of vast regions of space in which extremely small particles called electrons move around the atom's nucleus. Further research revealed that fundamentally it is energy – the force of electrical attraction between the nucleus of each atom and the electrons travelling around it – which forms the basis not only of all solids, liquids and gases, but also of all living things and the biological processes that bring them into existence.

Human beings are essentially composed of and subject to the same basic energy forces as all animate and inanimate matter, and the entire Universe is united by the principle force of energy.

ALBERT EINSTEIN
Revolutionising modern thinking, Einstein discovered that every particle of matter is charged with electromagnetic energy.

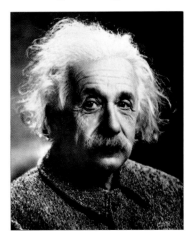

Einstein's theory of relativity demonstrated that this energy was constantly dynamic, constantly changing matter into different forms and states.

PARALLELS WITH EASTERN RELIGIONS

In reaching this radical new understanding of the world, the new physics has been observed to have many parallels with Eastern thought and religion. In 1974 physicist Fritjof Capra was the first to explore these parallels in his best-selling book, *The Tao of Physics*. He argued that religions such as Buddhism, Hinduism and Taoism all place dynamic energy at the centre of the Universe, and see all things – food, the seasons, people, even the arrangement of furniture in our houses – as being imbued with and subject to dynamic, constantly changing energy, and that this was just one of many similarities between modern physics and ancient religions.

The complexity of modern physics is daunting; yet the more we learn about what affects our own energy levels, the more these theories seem to make sense. Our fluctuating energy levels cannot be explained by any one factor: all the forces and elements we interact with, from the people we meet, the emotions we experience, the seasons, and the food we eat, will all influence our level of energy. The holistic way of looking at health is embodied in Ayurvedic medicine and traditional Chinese medicine.

THE HUMAN BODY AND ENERGY

Your energy relates directly to the amount and type of food you eat. This link has always been apparent to even the most basic societies, although exactly how food was digested and energy gained was not so obvious. The ancient Greeks were the first to experiment with digestion and the physician Galen calculated digestion rates in the stomach, but wrongly believed that the nourishment from food was absorbed, transformed into a milky liquid and passed into the liver, where it was imbued with a natural spirit, making energy.

The Renaissance brought in a new wave of medical research and Italian academics proposed that the digestive system worked like a machine, although the soul was still named as the driving force behind it. It was not until the early 19th century that the US

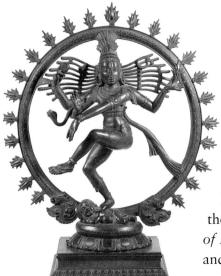

SHIVA
This statuette depicts Shiva, the Hindu god symbolising unity of opposites.

HEALTHY DIET
Energy comes from the food that we eat. The better quality fuel we consume, in the form of fresh fruit and vegetables and complex carbohydrates, the higher our energy levels.

surgeon, William Beaumont, made headway into understanding the digestive processes. His research formed the basis for the work of the French scientist, Claude Bernard, who made the breakthrough discovery that all food was absorbed into the blood and taken to the liver, where it was transformed into sugar and glycogen which could be used to form energy.

The vital role that oxygen plays in food digestion was first discovered in the 18th century by the Irish scientist Robert Boyle. Then, early in the 19th century the Italian physicist and priest, Lazzaro Spallanzani, reached the conclusion that the transformation of food into energy took place in every tissue in the body as oxygen was transformed into carbon dioxide.

The exact process by which each cell produces energy was not discovered until after the Second World War when powerful microscopes and research instruments allowed scientists to observe the action of cells for the first time. The role of hormones (the name is derived from the Greek word 'to excite') in controlling metabolism and energy production was first identified in the 18th century, but the individual hormones and their functions were not established until the 20th century.

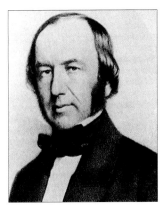

CLAUDE BERNARD
The great medic Claude Bernard made important advances in the fields of digestion and energy, hormones and metabolism.

THE HUMAN MIND AND ENERGY

Our understanding of how the mind affects energy has developed more slowly. The ancient Greeks recognised the importance of the brain as the centre of intellectual life and the seat of the soul. Some philosophers thought that sleep occurred thanks to a temporary retreat of blood from the brain, and that death indicated a permanent departure. Diseases of the brain, such as epilepsy, were known as 'sacred' diseases, and the feelings were believed to have sprung from the brain. The physician Galen described an 'animal spirit' coming from the brain that was concerned with intellectual activities, sensation and movement.

During the Renaissance and Enlightenment philosophers further analysed brain functioning and how the brain interacts with the nervous system and metabolism. However, the human psyche and thought processes – how we feel, think and decide – were not fully investigated until the early 20th century when

PSYCHOTHERAPY
Research has proven that positive emotional experiences and an optimistic mental attitude can dramatically improve energy levels.

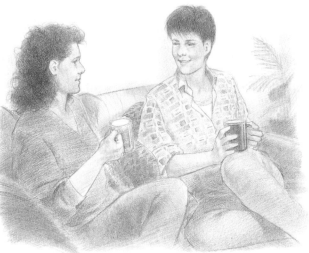

Sigmund Freud dared to analyse the human mind. The conclusion of Freud's research – namely that each person reacts to situations according to his or her own personal experience and physical and emotional needs – led to a surge in psychiatric and neurochemical analysis. It is now known that the mind plays an enormous role in the health and energy of the individual, through both hormone secretions in the brain and thoughts and feelings, and how they influence one another. Further research is needed to understand these processes more fully. However, today it is clear that patients with energy problems often benefit from psychotherapy or stress relief to help them to deal with their problems and address any hidden emotional agenda.

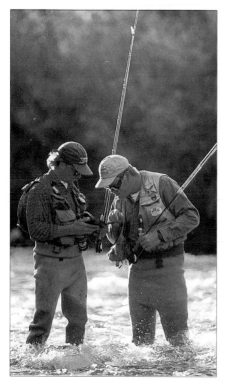

POSITIVE RELATIONSHIPS
Sharing positive energies with others and avoiding negative feelings can help you to stay happy and energised.

CREATING A HIGH-ENERGY LIFESTYLE

Whether you are suffering from sporadic tiredness, a general lack of energy, or have a more serious condition affecting your vitality, you can make a number of simple adjustments to your lifestyle that will dramatically improve your get-up-and-go. *Energise Your Life* will help you to identify and make the most appropriate changes for maximising your energy levels. Every aspect of how and where energy is required, produced and used in the body is covered in detail, enabling you to understand how you can better maintain your vim and vigour.

Chapter 1 looks at how energy is produced. Every person has different energy levels and food needs, depending on his or her energy expenditure. Your hormonal status, including your sexual hormones, play a large part in energy balance and understanding your body can help you to adapt to hormonal changes, such as those that accompany menstruation or old age.

Chapter 2 investigates natural energy sources and how they have been used in certain cultures and for energy therapies. Chapter 3 covers potential energy drainers in your life, such as sleeping problems, caffeine and emotional disruption.

Chapter 4 considers healthy nutrition, focusing on the nutrients that you need for energy and how to prevent debilitating deficiencies. Exercises for physical and mental energy are covered in Chapter 5, including relaxation techniques. Chapter 6 describes the more serious conditions that are associated with low energy, such as ME and anaemia, and what you can do about them.

ARE YOU MAKING THE MOST OF YOUR ENERGY POTENTIAL?

How often do you feel tired and unwilling to do the things that you usually enjoy? Most people experience periods of low energy – some more than others – but there is much you can do to maintain your zest. Understanding how you gain and expend energy can help you to make the most of your health and vitality, allowing you to pursue your goals and achieve the things that you want.

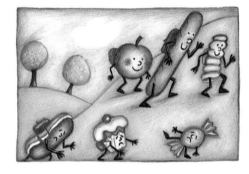

Q **ARE YOU GETTING THE RIGHT QUANTITIES AND TYPES OF FOOD?**
Your primary source of energy is the food that you eat, but much depends on how well it is digested. For maximum energy potential, the best foods are complex carbohydrates, such as wholegrain bread, pasta and rice, and plenty of fruit, vegetables, nuts and beans. Sugar and foods high in sugar, such as cakes and sweets, offer nothing but a 'sugar rush' which only leaves you feeling even more tired and lacking in blood sugar a few hours later. A healthy balanced diet is the best grounding for high energy levels (see Chapter 4).

Q **ARE YOU GETTING ENOUGH NUTRIENTS?**
Nutrients play a crucial role in the functioning of everyday bodily processes, including food absorption, energy production and proper mental functioning. If your energy levels are low, you may not be getting all the minerals and vitamins that you need in your diet. You can rectify this by adjusting your diet to include foods rich in nutrients, or by taking supplements if necessary. You may also suffer from mild nutrient deficiencies if your body is not absorbing the nutrients from food properly. This may be caused by other nutritional deficiencies, drinking alcohol or smoking, or by a more serious condition. Chapter 4 details the essential nutrients for health and energy.

Q **DO YOU FEEL OUT OF BREATH IF YOU RUN UP THE STAIRS?**
Your body becomes more energised the more that it is used – so build more exercise into your routine (see Chapter 5). Taking regular exercise and raising your heartbeat for over 20 minutes three times a week will give you the get-up-and-go that you need for your everyday life.

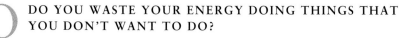

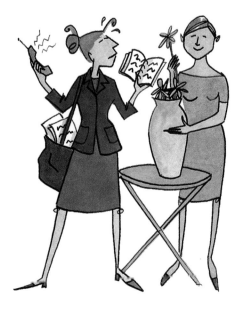

Q DO YOU WASTE YOUR ENERGY DOING THINGS THAT YOU DON'T WANT TO DO?

You may be wasting your energy on things that are not important. Worrying about unimportant issues, getting upset or distracted by others, feeling guilty about your actions or overburdening stress are all negative feelings which can drain your energy before you get a chance to do the things that are important to you. Listening to your feelings, sorting the negative from the positive and not allowing unnecessary worries to drain you physically can help you to find more energy. Motivating yourself with new challenges, or rewarding yourself when you meet your own personal goals, can work miracles in finding new reserves of untapped energy. Taking up new pastimes or hobbies, or maybe a change of job, can help you to channel your energy and challenge yourself with new experiences.

Q DO YOU THINK YOU MAY HAVE A MORE SERIOUS MEDICAL PROBLEM?

Fatigue is a symptom of most medical conditions as the body attempts to counteract the effects of an illness, disease or deficiency. This means that locating and treating the cause of fatigue can be difficult, although many tests can be performed to try to diagnose specific conditions so that they can be properly treated. The main physical problems associated with fatigue are discussed in Chapter 6, which also examines chronic fatigue syndrome or ME. For many conditions dietary changes, herbal supplements and other complementary therapies can do a great deal to relieve symptoms, although you should always consult your doctor first if you are suffering from fatigue for no apparent reason.

Q DO YOU GET ENOUGH REST AND RELAXATION?

If you feel tired, do you rest properly, or merely sit down and worry about your problems? Proper rest and relaxation means resting your body, your mind and your emotions, giving yourself a complete break from life's ups and downs. This can be achieved by mental relaxation exercises, such as meditation, yoga and chi kung (see Chapter 5) which aim to raise you above day-to-day worries. A good night's sleep, without the use of pills, is fundamental, and if you have trouble sleeping or wake up often, you might like to consider the action steps described in Chapter 3. Sleep is one of the first things that people skip if they have a busy schedule, although they rarely consider the broader effects that lack of sleep has on their lives and energy levels.

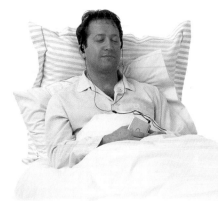

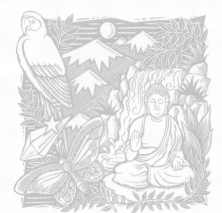

CHAPTER 1

ENERGY AND THE INDIVIDUAL

Every movement and body process is fuelled by energy. It is energy that enables you to think, feel, work, play and stay healthy. The energy for life comes from food and drink, which the individual cells in the body break down and convert into a form that can be used for living. But other factors – both internal and external – affect the amount of energy you have at different stages of your life.

WHAT IS ENERGY?

Energy makes all activity possible; anything that moves or grows uses energy to do so. When energy is at a peak, you will not only feel vital, your general health will also be excellent.

Energy forms the basis of our lives. All life on earth is based on systems of energy-giving life, providing light and warmth, enabling growth, movement and action. Energy is needed for everything we do: from lighting and heating our homes and workplaces to transporting us and feeding us. Energy is also the basis of the body's own systems: energy keeps us alive and functioning efficiently and effectively.

Ultimately all energy on earth, including the energy that sustains our bodies, derives either directly or indirectly from the sun. For example, fuels such as coal and oil were formed millions of years ago from vegetation. When oil or coal is burnt as fuel the energy released is derived from the sun's rays absorbed by prehistoric trees and plants. In the same way our own energy supply is derived from the energy from the sun absorbed by the plants we eat today. Plants use the light from the sun to make sugars from carbon dioxide and water.

THE LAWS OF ENERGY

Because energy is so all-encompassing in our lives, it is difficult to define precisely. However, scientists have determined a number of laws about how energy works. These laws can be applied to understanding how energy works in our own bodies.

First, energy cannot be created from nothing. Things do not become 'energised' by themselves, they are acted upon by other energy forces. For example, a toy car doesn't start to move by itself: either it is wound-up using an internal slow-release spring, or it is run by a battery utilising chemical energy, or the child uses his or her own energy to move it. Although this may seem obvious, it is a point many people forget when they are

under pressure from work or family commitments. If you eat poorly or irregularly, and take inadequate rest, you are ultimately asking your body to create energy from nothing and will end up tired and run-down.

The second law of energy is that it can be changed into various forms. For example, winding up a spring in a clockwork car creates 'potential' energy. Until the spring unwinds the car is apparently without energy, but the spring holds the potential to make the car move. Once the car is moving it is described as having 'kinetic' energy, the name applied to the energy of all moving objects. Other kinds of energy include chemical energy. An example of this is the process of photosynthesis whereby chemical molecules in plants convert light energy from the sun into sugars. Similarly, as humans the energy we receive and use undergoes changes in form. The food we eat contains chemical energy in the form of plant and animal sugars. These sugars may then be transformed into heat energy, maintaining our body at the correct temperature; some energy may become kinetic energy as we take a walk, for example; and some energy is stored in our cells as potential energy, to be released as our body requires.

The third energy principle is that of conservation. Expressed simply, this means that although energy can be changed into different forms the amount of energy after the change is equal to the amount of energy at the start. So if we eat foods of low nutritional value our bodies will only be able to produce a similar low level of energy, and we will lack vitality.

Of course the human body is far more complex than a plant. Our energy levels are also affected by the intricate workings of the brain. Many people underestimate the draining effects of prolonged emotional stress, for example. Your body responds to

FEELING ENERGY
Your energy levels are the result of many factors: the air that you breathe, the food that you eat, as well as your emotional state.

16

stress with the physical reactions of increased heart rate, breathing rate and higher blood pressure. Your liver also releases energy-giving sugars to boost your general energy levels. This response causes a huge drain in your energy supplies. Even though our emotions may seem quite separate to our physical processes, in fact they have a very real impact on bodily health, especially on hormone secretion and energy.

We are also affected by external energy forces apart from the food we eat. For example, medical science utilises forms of energy forces to treat illnesses and diseases. Radiation therapy uses electromagnetic energy to destroy cancerous cells in the body. However, many complementary and alternative therapists believe that we are influenced by energy in a more integral way. Some see individual people as having their own energy fields that interact on a constant basis with all the energy forces of nature. For example, many Eastern philosophies see a change in energy levels relating to the change in seasons, and believe we should adjust our lifestyle and behaviour to correspond with these external changes.

Perhaps the crucial point to remember when thinking about your energy level is that energy is all-encompassing. Energy is influenced by forces both external and internal; the key to good health lies in finding a harmonious balance in the forces that influence our lives.

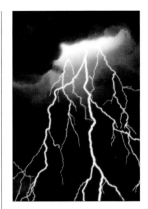

LIGHTNING
Energy is released from highly charged particles in the atmosphere.

FACTORS THAT AFFECT ENERGY

Taking time to plan your life can help you to manage your energy better and control the factors around you which are affecting your energy levels. Confusion, stress and not knowing what you want are the greatest of all drains on your energy. Take steps towards conquering them by making a list of the things that you like and you want to see happening in your future. If you recognise the factors that affect your energy, you can work out ways to counter them and help to realise your potential energy levels.

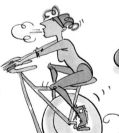

Sleep and rest
It is essential to rest properly in order to restore your body. During sleep, your body and mind have time to relax and unwind – you may be unaware of the stress you have experienced.

The seasons
The climate and weather can influence your energy levels. The lack of sunshine in the winter can leave you feeling tired, and you need extra energy boosts in this season.

Relationships
Positive relations with those around you can help you to feel happy. Sharing a relationship with someone special can add an extra zest to your life.

Exercise
Regular exercise, raising your heartbeat for 20 minutes three times a week, boosts health and improves energy.

A healthy diet
Eating the nutrients that you need for proper body functioning and getting enough nourishment for energy are the crucial dietary factors for good energy and health.

Weight watching
Keeping your weight at a normal level boosts your health and energy. Carrying around more weight than you need only slows you down and tires you out.

Sex
A fulfilling and happy sex life is an important part of your personal and emotional health. It can also be fun and relaxing, enabling you to reaffirm a good relationship.

Fulfilling your potential
Recognising, pursuing and ultimately fulfilling your ambitions, goals and dreams can be one of the most difficult but rewarding challenges of your life. In order to live a happy, balanced and energised life, you must realise your potential and aim for the goals that you have set for yourself.

Environmental factors
Living in a healthy environment and setting aside time to enjoy the countryside and natural beauty of the world around you can help to boost your energy.

Light and colour
Living with the colours that help you to feel energised can boost your vitality. Light is an essential element in supplying energy not just for us but for all the life on the planet.

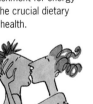

ENERGY AND YOUR BODY

Understanding the processes by which your body gains and expends energy will help you to recognise the factors that cause different people to have different energy levels.

The energy that powers your muscles and fuels your brain comes from what you eat. The process begins in your digestive system where the energy-giving nutrients are extracted from food and passed into your bloodstream. This complex procedure occurs at different rates throughout the day and according to your age, state of health and dietary needs, as well as the type of food that you are eating.

THE DIGESTIVE SYSTEM

Food is absorbed through the digestive system in a variety of ways, usually with the help of enzymes released by the body to help the breakdown of food. The food is eventually broken down into glucose which can be converted with oxygen into energy.

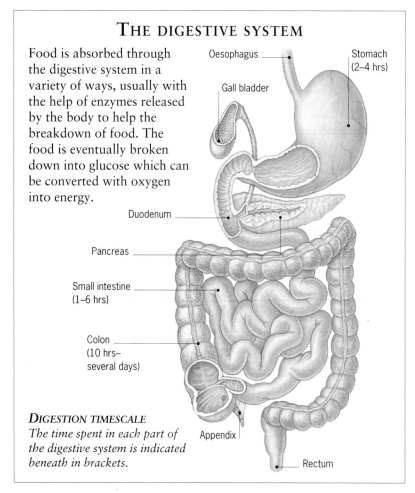

Oesophagus

Gall bladder

Stomach
(2–4 hrs)

Duodenum

Pancreas

Small intestine
(1–6 hrs)

Colon
(10 hrs–
several days)

Appendix

Rectum

DIGESTION TIMESCALE
The time spent in each part of the digestive system is indicated beneath in brackets.

THE DIGESTIVE SYSTEM

The digestive tract, also known as the alimentary canal, is like a continuous series of tubes, including the stomach, that extend right through the body from the mouth to the anus. In adults this tract is over 10 metres (33 feet) long. Different sections of this tube have different functions. Other important parts of the digestive system include the teeth, tongue and salivary glands, and the swallowing mechanism in the oesophagus (gullet). The liver and pancreas are situated in the abdomen. Digestion begins when you chew your food. The saliva begins the chemical breakdown of the food, because it contains an enzyme (a protein that speeds up chemical reactions) that converts starches to sugars.

When you swallow the food, a series of muscular contractions pushes it down your oesophagus, the tube that connects your throat to your stomach. Once in your stomach, the food is mixed with digestive juices that begin to break it down into its component nutrients. This process is aided by rhythmic movements of the stomach wall.

Some of the nutrients in the food – such as glucose and water – can be absorbed directly through the stomach wall and pass into the bloodstream for immediate use by your body, but most of them pass from your stomach into your small intestine. Digestion is completed there with the aid of digestive juices from the liver and pancreas, and the nutrients from food are absorbed into your bloodstream through the intestine wall.

By the time it leaves the small intestine and enters the large intestine (colon), almost all of the usable nutrients in the food have been removed from it. As it passes through the large intestine, bacteria living in the intestine decompose the food, a process that produces gas and some B-group vitamins. By the time the residue of the digested food is expelled from the body, it consists of about 75 per cent water and 25 per cent solids, composed mainly of undigested fibre, dead bacteria, fat, inorganic matter, and a small amount of protein.

BREAKING DOWN FOOD FOR ENERGY

The main sources of energy in food are carbohydrates (sugars and starches) and fats, but some energy also comes from proteins. Carbohydrates are found in foods such as bread, pasta, fruit, potatoes, rice and beans, and are built up from carbon, hydrogen and oxygen. The most basic forms of carbohydrate are the simple sugars called monosaccharides. These sugars, which include glucose, are the building blocks of the other carbohydrates. Then there are the disaccharides – more complex sugars consisting of pairs of monosaccharides – and the polysaccharides, or starches, which are made up of long chains of disaccharides.

Fats, from foods such as dairy products, vegetable oils, fish and meat, are also made up of carbon, hydrogen and oxygen, but these are combined in more complex ways than they are in carbohydrates to form the basic components of fat, which are called glycerol and fatty acids. Proteins – contained in meat, poultry, fish, beans and lentils – are even more complex, being built up from chains of amino acids consisting of carbon, hydrogen, oxygen and nitrogen.

In the digestive system, all carbohydrates are broken down into glucose, which passes into the bloodstream (as blood sugar) to be carried around the body as the principal energy source for use by muscles and cells. Fats are broken down into glycerol and fatty acids, and proteins into amino acids. These also enter the bloodstream, to be used for maintaining body tissue and for energy.

ENERGY TRANSFER

The energy that powers muscles and cells is chemical energy released when a substance called adenosine triphosphate (ATP) is

> **DID YOU KNOW?**
> When Henry VIII died aged 55 years, he was grossly overweight due to the abundant court feasts. As a result, he suffered from kidney disease, gout, circulatory disorders and a 'tortuously painful' leg ulcer which afflicted him throughout his later years.

Energy and activity

The more active you are, the harder your metabolism has to work to produce the energy you need. A man burns about 90 calories an hour while sitting, 120 when standing, 220 when walking, and 600 while running. A woman burns 70 calories an hour while sitting, 100 when standing, 180 when walking, and 420 while running.

AEROBIC AND ANAEROBIC ENERGY

During normal muscle use, including moderate exercise, the series of chemical reactions that convert food into energy for your muscles is an aerobic process, that is, it uses oxygen. The word *aerobic* comes from the Greek word for air. But when you exercise strenuously, your muscles use up oxygen (and glucose) faster than your bloodstream can supply it. When this happens, your muscles run out of energy and rapidly tire. This shortage of energy can be overcome by the action of a back-up chemical in the muscles – phosphorylcreatine. This chemical can supply energy when oxygen is in short supply, although only over a short period, such as for a sprint. Because this type of energy production uses no oxygen it is an *anaerobic* process.

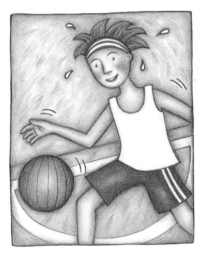

ANAEROBIC EXERCISE
Anaerobic exercise occurs when you exert yourself greatly for a short period, such as the burst of energy needed to sprint down a basketball court or run for a bus.

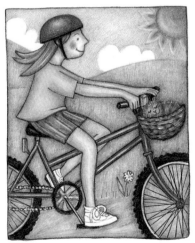

AEROBIC EXERCISE
Long bike rides, hill walking and jogging are all good examples of exercise that uses oxygen, utilising your lungs and heart and improving all-round fitness and health.

OBESITY AND ENERGY LEVELS

Obesity occurs when you are heavily overweight, usually defined as being over 30 per cent above the average weight for your height, according to the British Medical Association. The health problems linked with obesity include lack of physical fitness, depression and the impairment of the immune function. It also increases the risk of heart disease and high blood pressure. In many other conditions, such as non-insulin-dependent diabetes (see page 142), an overweight or obese sufferer is over five times more likely to die prematurely.

ENERGY REQUIREMENTS
People need to consume different levels of food to keep their energy supply in line with their expenditure. An active lifestyle needs to be fed, while a sedentary person would quickly become fat on the same diet.

broken down into a simpler substance, adenosine diphosphate (ADP). To keep this energy-producing process going, the ADP is converted back into ATP by the energy released when glucose is broken down and combined with oxygen in the bloodstream. This process allows energy to be released for movement and energy.

As well as delivering oxygen, the bloodstream collects carbon dioxide and water – the byproducts of the energy-producing process. These are taken away by red blood cells and by the plasma, the liquid part of the blood that carries the blood cells. This process is therefore dependent on the proper functioning of the blood, particularly the red blood cells, oxygen from the lungs, and glucose and fatty acids from food.

STORING ENERGY

Not all of the energy in the food you eat is required immediately, so your body needs some way of storing the surplus for later use. Surplus glucose, derived from carbohydrate foods, is converted into glycogen (a complex carbohydrate) which is stored in your muscles and liver. As the glucose in your bloodstream is used up to provide energy, glycogen is converted back into glucose and released into the bloodstream. Glycogen can also be made from protein and from the glycerol in fats; protein is first converted into amino acids and glucose.

When your glycogen stores are full, any surplus glucose and other energy-producing nutrients are stored as body fat. This fat can then be broken down into glycerol and fatty acids again when it is needed to provide energy. Body fat takes two forms, brown and white, and is stored in layers of cells under your skin, especially on the buttocks and around your kidneys and heart.

Brown fat, a kind of medium-term energy store, is the first to be used when your blood glucose levels are running low, for instance when you have been exercising hard or have not eaten for some time. White fat, the type

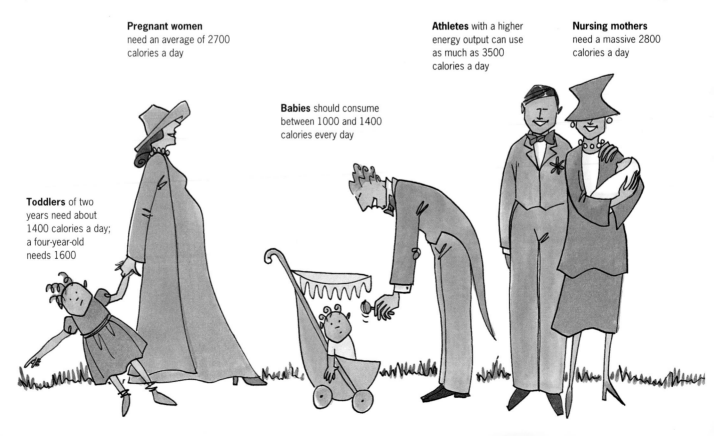

Pregnant women need an average of 2700 calories a day

Athletes with a higher energy output can use as much as 3500 calories a day

Nursing mothers need a massive 2800 calories a day

Babies should consume between 1000 and 1400 calories every day

Toddlers of two years need about 1400 calories a day; a four-year-old needs 1600

that causes obesity, is a long-term store where your body builds up energy reserves when the brown fat cells are full.

A healthy level of body fat is good as it protects the body against the cold and physical harm, and acts as a reserve store of energy. However, many people have a tendency to store too much fat, leading to the health problems associated with being overweight or obese.

METABOLISM

Metabolism consists of catabolic and anabolic processes. Catabolism takes place when energy is produced by the breaking down of complex substances into simpler ones, such as the breakdown of glucose into carbon dioxide and water. In contrast, anabolism uses energy to build up simple substances into more complex ones. For example, when amino acids – which are produced

from food proteins by catabolism – are reassembled into body-building proteins for making muscle tissue.

The amount of energy your metabolism produces over a given time is known as your metabolic rate. When you are resting your metabolism is just ticking over, producing the energy needed to sustain vital functions such as breathing, heartbeat, digestion and maintaining body temperature. The amount of energy you produce and use when you are resting is your basal metabolic rate (BMR), which varies according to age, height, weight, sex and other factors, such as pregnancy and breastfeeding a baby.

As soon as you start to move about, your metabolic rate increases to provide the extra energy you need. This increase is triggered by the action of hormones, such as adrenaline, insulin, steroids and thyroxine.

When your metabolic rate rises, your body responds by converting food or fat reserves into energy. If your intake and output of energy is about equal, then you will have a healthy weight. If you eat less than you need for energy, then you will lose weight. This is the basis of the concept of a calorie-controlled diet. If, on the other hand, you are eating more than you burn up, the excess energy will be stored as fat on your body. This happens often with people as they get older and become less active but do not reduce the amount of food they eat.

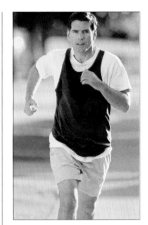

KEEPING ACTIVE
Regular aerobic exercise for 20 minutes or more improves your body's ability to produce energy.

DID YOU KNOW?

The 400-metre run is known to be one of the most difficult races because it is too long to run anaerobically, and yet too short to be an enduring aerobic exercise. Most runners use a combination of aerobic and anaerobic energy to cover the distance. When to begin the final sprint is considered a crucial and tactical point.

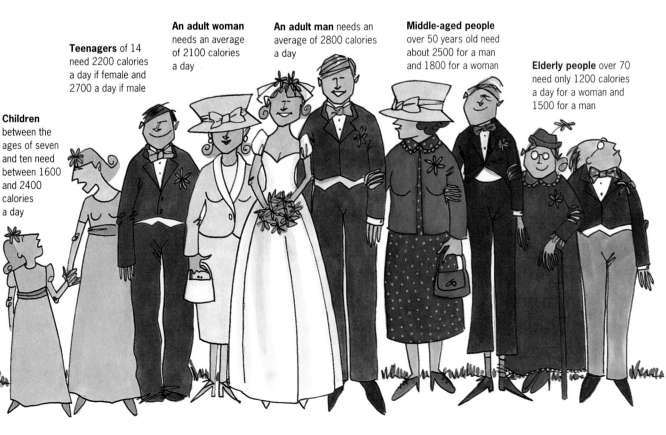

Children between the ages of seven and ten need between 1600 and 2400 calories a day

Teenagers of 14 need 2200 calories a day if female and 2700 a day if male

An adult woman needs an average of 2100 calories a day

An adult man needs an average of 2800 calories a day

Middle-aged people over 50 years old need about 2500 for a man and 1800 for a woman

Elderly people over 70 need only 1200 calories a day for a woman and 1500 for a man

GROWING NEEDS

Children require large amounts of food in comparison to their weight and height to enable them to grow and be active. Both calorie intake and protein needs rise steeply until the end of puberty when they level off once a balanced adult weight is reached. Boys usually need more food than girls in order to develop and maintain more tissue for muscle mass, and girls' requirements can decrease after puberty.

CALORIE INTAKE
Calories supply the energy-producing elements in your diet. They will be stored as fat if they are not used.

PROTEIN NEEDS
Protein is needed for growth and is also essential for the proper functioning of the body and for repair of tissues. It can also be used as a source of energy.

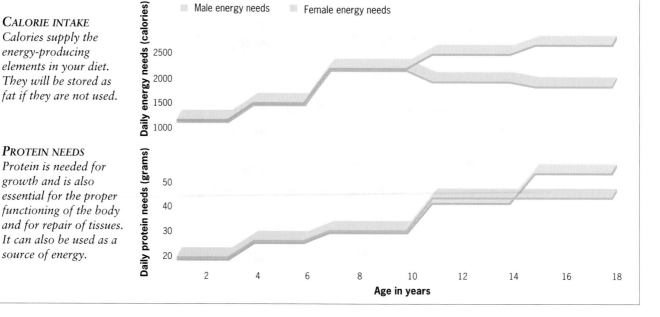

Male energy needs Female energy needs

Daily energy needs (calories)

2500
2000
1500
1000

Daily protein needs (grams)

50
40
30
20

2 4 6 8 10 12 14 16 18
Age in years

ENERGY REQUIREMENTS AND AGE

Children have a higher BMR than adults, mainly because they require more energy for growing, and their diet should include slightly more fat and sugar than an adult's diet. Children entering puberty and in their early teens have a lower BMR than younger ones, although calcium levels should be kept high as the bones are still growing. A diet high in nutrients is needed during the growth spurt at puberty. Girls in particular require large amounts of minerals and vitamins (but not necessarily calories), especially iron, magnesium and the vitamin B complexes, to help their bodies cope with the onset of menstruation. Boys, on the other hand, have rapidly growing muscle mass and height at this time and their calorie demands can be huge.

The BMR declines after puberty and usually continues to decline gently until middle age when the levels of energy begin to decrease more rapidly. Over the age of 50, people experience a reduction in body tissue, particularly affecting muscle mass and bone density, and a decrease in the efficiency of the organs. More fat will develop, in combination with a reduction in appetite, and there is a trend towards change in the hormone levels affecting all glands, particularly the thyroid (see page 140). This is a gradual process, and its rate of progression varies widely; some individuals appear to be more healthy and not as affected as others.

Modern research has shown that there is no one single factor which brings about the cellular changes of ageing, although a poor

ENERGY BOOST

Visit your local swimming pool for relaxation and exercise. Water provides a supportive environment for your muscles and joints, enabling you to take exercise without putting a strain on any part of your body. It can be particularly beneficial if you are recovering from an accident or injury and cannot exercise in the normal way. If you cannot swim, you can float and stretch your body in the water and enjoy its therapeutic benefits, or use a float to learn how to swim.

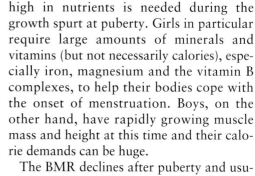

Does your lifestyle maximise your energy?

The energy that you have depends to a large degree on your diet and lifestyle. Not getting enough rest, too much stress, a poor diet and no exercise are the major factors that lead to energy loss, weight gain and poor health. Answer this questionnaire to find out whether your lifestyle is making it difficult for your body to get the energy it needs. Write the answer to each question on a piece of paper, then count how many a's, b's and c's you have. Read what each means in the key below for tips on how to improve your lifestyle.

How many times a week do you take exercise?

a) Three or more
b) Once or twice
c) Never

How many portions of fruit or vegetables, excluding potatoes, do you eat every day?

a) 5 or more
b) 2 to 4
c) 0 or 1

How do you feel about your weight?

a) About right
b) Could lose half a stone
c) Could lose more than a stone

Do you ever feel that you cannot be bothered or lack the motivation to do something that you have planned to do?

a) Rarely
b) Sometimes
c) Often

Do you need caffeine to get you going when you wake up in the morning?

a) Rarely or sometimes
b) Often
c) Every day

Do you smoke cigarettes or any tobacco products?

a) Rarely
b) Sometimes
c) Often

Are you stressed or anxious, or feel that you have lost control of your life?

a) Rarely
b) Sometimes
c) Often

Do you feel relaxed and unflustered?

a) Most of the time
b) Sometimes or often
c) Rarely

Do you lie in bed in the morning because you don't want, or don't feel able, to get up?

a) Rarely
b) Sometimes
c) Often

Do you feel that you waste your energy on things of no benefit?

a) Rarely
b) Sometimes
c) Often

Do you ever experience a shortness of breath?

a) Only after exercise
b) After any physical exertion
c) Most of the time

How many units of alcohol do you consume on average each day?

a) 0–2
b) 3–5
c) Over 6

Do you get the sleep that you need?

a) Usually
b) Sometimes or often
c) Rarely

How many portions of fried food, or sweets, cakes and biscuits do you consume on average every day?

a) 0–2
b) 3–5
c) Over 6

How often do you take time off to relax properly and forget your worries?

a) Twice a week at least
b) Once a week or fortnight
c) Once a month or less

Mostly a's: You are living a healthy lifestyle and should have no problems in finding the energy that you need to do the things that you want to do. Make a note of any questions that you did not score well on and watch out for those problems that are holding you back. Keeping your lifestyle healthy is not always easy, especially in times of trouble, and it is always important to take time off to relax properly. Relaxation techniques can be found in Chapter 5. Ensuring that you are eating a healthy diet and boosting your energy with vitamin-rich fresh fruit and vegetables may also help you retain your health.

Mostly b's: Although your lifestyle is relatively healthy, there are still a number of ways that it can be improved. Paying a little more attention to your health will increase the quality of your life, giving you the rest and energy for all the things that you want to do. Making sure that you are eating a proper diet is an easy way to enhance your health, and it can be delicious too (see Chapter 4). Cutting down on caffeine can also help your energy levels.

Mostly c's: You need to pay more attention to your health and lifestyle, and adjustments need to be made if you want to increase your energy levels. Regular exercise can boost your health substantially (see pages 112–18), and ensuring that you get enough sleep to recuperate properly rebalances your system (see pages 54–7). Cutting out smoking and alcohol may also be of help, especially in the mornings when energy may be hard to find.

THE GROWTH SPURT

As children grow into adults they experience a growth spurt, usually around the time of puberty when the body is preparing for reproduction.

During this time, the child will need more food for energy and growth, particularly boys, whose growth spurt is greater, and slightly later, than girls'.

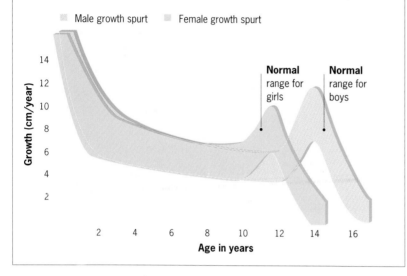

Male growth spurt   Female growth spurt

Growth (cm/year)

Normal range for girls

Normal range for boys

Age in years

coordinate the functions of your body's cells and organs. They are secreted by the glands which respond to a number of stimuli.

The more important hormones in energy metabolism include thyroxine, insulin, glucagon and adrenaline. Thyroxine, produced in the thyroid glands, controls the metabolic rate and energy production. Insulin and glucagon are produced by the pancreas, and adrenaline by the adrenal glands, which are situated on top of the kidneys. Together, these hormones control the production and use of glucose and glycogen, which is synthesised from surplus glucose in your bloodstream and stored in your liver and muscles. When your blood-glucose levels need boosting, the glycogen is converted back into glucose.

Insulin and glucagon together regulate the amount of glucose in the blood to keep it close to its optimum level. When your blood-glucose level falls, either because more glucose is being used to produce energy or because you have not eaten for some time, glucagon stimulates the breakdown of the glycogen reserves within the body into glucose. This breakdown is accelerated if necessary by the action of thyroxine or adrenaline when extra energy is needed.

Insulin has the opposite effect. When your blood-glucose level rises above its normal level, as it does after eating a meal, insulin

diet, environmental factors and lack of exercise can all have an effect.

THE INFLUENCE OF HORMONES

Hormones are substances that circulate in the bloodstream. They act as chemical messengers, carrying signals that control and

THE ENDOCRINE SYSTEM

The endocrine system is a complicated network of hormone-producing glands. The hypothalamus in the brain stimulates the pituitary gland which in turn regulates most of the other hormones of the body. It stimulates the adrenals, thyroid, pigment-producing skin cells, and gonads, which control the sex hormones. It also secretes growth hormone, antidiuretic hormone, prolactin, which stimulates the growth and development of the breasts, and oxytocin, which is important during pregnancy.

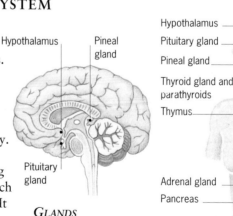

Hypothalamus   Pineal gland

Pituitary gland

Hypothalamus
Pituitary gland
Pineal gland
Thyroid gland and parathyroids
Thymus
Adrenal gland
Pancreas
Ovaries

GLANDS
Hormonal glands are positioned around the body and within the major organs. They secrete their specific hormones directly into the bloodstream.

stimulates the production of glycogen to mop up the excess, and when your glycogen stores are full it will initiate the conversion of glucose to body fat. It also plays a key role in the production of energy by enabling the transport of glucose into the cells from the bloodstream – without insulin this would not be possible.

A temporary low level of blood-glucose often happens if you miss a meal. This can make you feel lacking in energy, irritable, and unable to concentrate, but these symptoms soon disappear when you eat a meal, or even a snack, and your blood-glucose level returns to normal.

A serious cause of low blood-glucose is the presence of excess insulin in the bloodstream. This can happen to people with insulin-dependent diabetes, a metabolic disorder caused by the failure of the pancreas to produce enough insulin. To counteract this disorder, insulin-dependent diabetics have to inject themselves with insulin at least once a day in order to prevent their blood-glucose levels becoming too high, while also eating enough carbohydrate to stop them becoming too low. If they take too much insulin or not enough carbohydrate, their blood-glucose levels can become dangerously low. This can be quickly remedied by taking a sugary food or drink, but if ignored it can lead to unconsciousness.

Hormonal balance plays a major role in vitality. Keeping your body healthy and regularly active can help to achieve an equilibrium between the chemical hormones being produced by the body and those being used.

Anything that reduces stress and infection and promotes good sleep and exercise will clearly have a beneficial effect on our general health and energy levels, especially with increasing age. Both exercise and forms of relaxation therapy appear to have direct effects on hormones which influence our energy levels. Researchers at James Cook University in Australia studied the relationship between hormones and mood changes in 11 elite runners and 12 highly trained meditators who were matched for age, sex and personality. Each performed their specialised activity for 30 minutes and their hormone changes were registered over a period of time. The findings were that both activities stimulated similar hormonal responses, in addition to a general lift in mood. The hormone cortisol, which has

THE HORMONES

The hormones play an important part in the functioning of the human body. If they are out of balance or undergoing a process of change, the body will react differently and will not be able to utilise energy effectively.

LOCATION	HORMONES PRODUCED	EFFECTS
Hypothalamus	Regulating hormones	Regulates other glands
Pituitary gland	Growth hormone Prolactin	Growth, metabolism Breast development
Brain	Endorphins	Painkilling and relaxing
Pineal gland	Melatonin	Synchronises biorhythms
Thyroid glands	Thyroxine	Metabolic rate
Adrenal glands	Adrenaline, noradrenaline Cortisol	Prepares for stress Hormone regulation
Pancreas	Insulin, glucagon	Regulates blood-sugar level
Ovaries	Oestrogen, progesterone	Menstruation, pregnancy, female sexual characteristics
Testes	Testosterone	Male sexual characteristics

been found to be significant in energy function, was higher in most participants at the end of their activity. This suggests that both of these practices can provide a boost in energy levels, and there is a growing use of meditation in fatigue relief.

continued on page 28

COSMIC ENERGY FORCES: *The Planets*

The planets have played a major role in theories of cosmic forces. The Greeks and Romans viewed the planets as gods and gave each a power. Mars is the god of war, for example, and Venus is the goddess of love, born out of the waves at Paphos in Cyprus. There are nine known planets in our solar system, although some astronomers suspect that there may be more. The planets form the central basis for biodynamic theory, which uses their natural guidance to understand the patterns of nature. The theory is used mostly within an agricultural context.

25

The Endocrinologist

Specialising in hormone disorders, an endocrinologist can help you to locate any hormone or glandular problems that may be affecting your energy levels and preventing you from being active. Endocrinologists can also help with hormone changes.

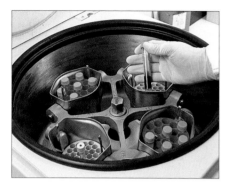

TESTING FOR HORMONE DISORDERS
A number of tests are used to check your hormone balance. Some can be performed by the endocrinologist, although others require specialised laboratory analysis.

The endocrinologist aims to investigate and rebalance the endocrine system – the network of glands involved in the production of hormones – and the factors that stimulate them. The hormones affect every function of your body, influencing energy levels from the very site of energy production, and any imbalance results in a lack of energy, as well as a number of knock-on effects and symptoms of poor health.

Origins

The pituitary gland has been recognised for its importance in brain function since the ancient Greek philosopher Aristotle proposed that a serum was emitted from the gland, influencing body processes. However, endocrinology has only recently become more properly understood. Guesses throughout the 19th century that the source of diabetes lay in the pancreas led to the discovery of glycogen by Claude Bernard in the 1850s, although insulin was not discovered until the 1920s by two Canadian physiologists, Frederick Banting and Charles Best. The first hormone to be properly isolated was secretin in 1902 by English physicians William Bayliss and Ernest Starling. Much of the work of the US surgeon Harvey Cushing, who greatly advanced neurosurgery in the 1930s, focused on the

pituitary gland. He suggested that 'the pituitary is the conductor of the endocrine orchestra', paving the way for further hormone research and developments in treatment.

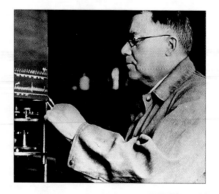

DR WALTER CANNON
Working as a doctor in the US in the 1930s, Cannon made great advances in the understanding of hormones and the mental state. His results and conclusions marked a major breakthrough in endocrinology.

What qualifications does an endocrinologist have?
An endocrinologist will have trained as a doctor and then specialised in endocrinology. A course takes at least five years of study, and the competition for places on an endocrinology course is tough. Following training, a doctor may begin to practise as a professional endocrinologist immediately.

When are patients referred to an endocrinologist?
A doctor will refer a patient to an endocrinologist if there is sufficient reason to suspect a problem with the hormone system. Common symptoms that may suggest an endocrine disorder include fatigue, inexplicable weight change, depression, anxiety or mood swings, change in skin and hair condition, diarrhoea or constipation, menstrual disorders, increased urinary output, and swelling of the glands, particularly those in the neck. The doctor will usually exclude more common or simple disorders before referral to an endocrinologist.

What will take place during a consultation?
The endocrinologist takes blood and urine tests to examine the levels of different hormones in the system. The results will reveal any discrepancies, which can then be treated. The treatment may be given by the endocrinologist, but sometimes the patient is referred back to his or her doctor with the

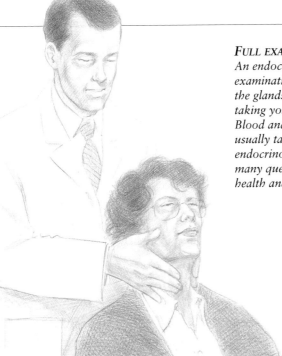

FULL EXAMINATION
An endocrinological examination includes feeling the glands, the pulse and taking your blood pressure. Blood and urine samples are usually taken for analysis. The endocrinologist will also ask many questions about your health and lifestyle.

to a drain on energy levels and an inability to live a normal life. The efficient working of the thyroid gland is essential for retaining healthy metabolic levels, and an endocrinologist can effectively diagnose and treat imbalances and restore health and vitality. Insulin disorders causing diabetes mellitus prevent glucose from being converted into energy, and insulin injections or dietary measures can help to normalise the energy balance. Hormones affecting the brain can also be rebalanced, including those that cause depression, anxiety and other debilitating psychological conditions which sap a person's motivation.

Where does an endocrinologist practise?
Endocrinology departments are usually found in the larger hospitals, although smaller hospitals that specialise in reproductive, digestive or psychological disorders often have endocrinologist units to help with hormonal disorders.

test results for further care. Other symptoms and your health history, including your emotional health, will be taken into consideration when deciding on the treatment, which may involve hormone replacement drugs, lifestyle changes, dietary measures or other treatments.

What are the most common conditions that an endocrinologist treats?
Thyroid disorders and diabetes mellitus are common problems that need to be diagnosed and treated by an endocrinologist. An analysis of the hypothalamus-pituitary system is also carried out on those with depressed energy levels. Some endocrinologists specialise in locating hormonal problems involving low energy and related disorders, such as myalgic encephalomyelitis (ME, see pages 150–3). Many of the more common hormonal problems, such as menstrual disorders, imbalances caused by the menopause, and prostate problems, are usually treated by a doctor or specialist of the reproductive organs.

How can an endocrinologist help to boost energy levels?
Hormonal complications come in a variety of forms, almost all leading

WHAT YOU CAN DO AT HOME

Some hormone problems can be countered at home by taking dietary precautions. Many minerals and vitamins can play a role in keeping you feeling normal through difficult hormonal changes.

For example, many people have a problem maintaining their sex drive after the hormonal changes that occur following middle age, affecting their sense of well-being and energy levels. This can be countered to an extent by eating a healthy and balanced diet, which gives you all the nutrients that you need. Zinc levels are considered particularly important in sexual activity: when your zinc levels are low, your blood histamine levels are also low, which may make it more difficult to reach orgasm. Since the refining processes remove 80 per cent of the zinc contents from cereals and grains, it is

important to choose foods that keep your zinc intake high. Good sources include oysters, clams, sardines and other seafood, seeds, nuts, root ginger, red meat and offal.

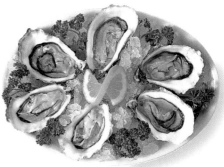

THE ULTIMATE APHRODISIAC
The ancient Greeks celebrated oysters for their aphrodisiac qualities, and their reputation remains to this day. Oysters contain high levels of important nutrients, encouraging a good sex life.

EFFECTS OF LOW ENERGY

Low energy can produce the following effects on a sufferer:

▶ *Inactivity.*

▶ *Intolerance to cold.*

▶ *Irritability.*

▶ *Depression or anxiety.*

▶ *Poor skin and hair condition.*

▶ *Prone to illness.*

CULTURAL FACTORS
Living conditions and lifestyle in different cultures may produce different energy demands. This woman is carrying her baby as she works, and she is also responsible for breast-feeding, and so will need a greater amount of energy in her diet than a woman of similar age in a leisured society.

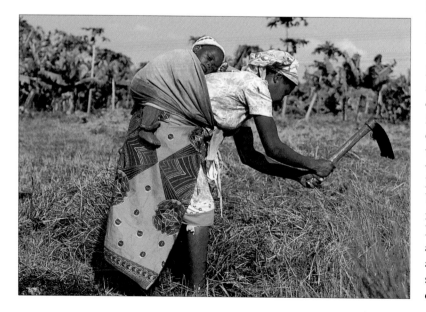

HORMONAL CHANGES

Hormonal changes affect everyone throughout their lives and can have serious effects on metabolism and energy levels. Mostly changes occur as the body alters with age or need, such as at the menopause. However, many changes cannot be explained so easily and may result from illness, stress or, sometimes, no apparent reason at all. The endocrine system – the network of glands releasing hormones into the bloodstream – may be affected by a number of factors, including emotional and mental processes.

The hormone condition most often linked with fatigue is thyroid disease, or a change in the hormone thyroxine, which is needed to stimulate your metabolism. A lack of thyroxine – hypothyroidism or myxoedema – can lead to lethargy, weight gain and muscular problems, and can also slow thinking and mental development in children. It can be easily treated with thyroid hormone replacement treatments.

The adrenal glands are responsible for the production of adrenaline, the hormone that causes blood to flow faster and the body to respond quickly to challenging situations. An excess of adrenaline and its related hormone, noradrenaline, results in high blood pressure, increased activity, anxiety and, in the long run, fatigue.

Another important hormone that influences energy level is cortisol. This is released from the adrenal cortex and is regulated by a complicated feedback mechanism involving both the hypothalamus and the pituitary gland. Low levels of cortisol can result in profound lethargy which is reversible on hormone replacement treatment.

Hormones concerned with reproduction can also cause energy imbalances. Changes in hormone levels during the menstrual cycle can seriously affect energy, and also during menopause. Pregnancy brings about probably the greatest changes in hormones experienced in a woman's life. Male hormones, especially testosterone, can play a major role in a man's energy levels.

GENETIC FACTORS

Genetics may be a factor in how much energy a person has. Abnormalities that can influence a person's energy may be present at birth or may not become apparent until middle or old age. Common diseases in which there is probably some genetic predisposition, such as diabetes mellitus and thyroid disease, have a pronounced effect on metabolism with resultant abnormal energy expenditure. The Pima Indians of South America have a genetic predisposition to develop diabetes, for example.

CULTURAL FACTORS

Food energy is usually stored as fat, and the fat stores in people differ widely throughout the world, depending on food supply and climate. As modern society, particularly in highly developed countries, is characterised by abundant food and labour-saving devices, such as cars, there is a tendency towards being overweight. Energy levels are greatly affected by fat levels as being overweight or obese lowers mobility and greatly increases the likelihood of energy-draining diseases, such as diabetes, hypertension, heart disease, arthritis and other illnesses.

Energy expenditure is also modified by how an individual is brought up and by social customs. Psychological, social and cultural factors, including race and religion, influence diet and hence individual energy expenditure. Different cultures have traditional ways of preparing and eating food that can make a great impact on energy and health. In Britain our diet is still dominated by fried foods, although more healthy cooking techniques are becoming more prevalent. It is estimated that 13 per cent of men and 16 per cent of women are obese, although a huge 43 per cent of men and some 24 per cent of women are overweight, causing many energy and health problems.

WOMEN AND ENERGY

Women usually experience more changes in their energy levels and metabolism throughout life than men, caused mainly by hormonal changes associated with menstruation and pregnancy.

Experiencing complicated hormonal changes every month with menstruation, women often find themselves feeling out of sorts and fatigued for no apparent reason. Realising and understanding the difficulties can allow you to boost your energy by eating a balanced diet, exercising properly and taking precautions so as not to drain your energy during the times when you need it most.

PREMENSTRUAL SYNDROME

Most women are affected to some extent by the hormonal changes associated with their menstrual cycle, although the severity varies enormously, having little impression on some and a more severe effect on others. Premenstrual syndrome (PMS) is caused by the series of hormonal changes that occur from eight to two days before menstruation. It is characterised by mood changes, irritability, food craving, behavioural changes and a lack of energy. Metabolic changes in severe PMS are quite marked and there is often swelling of the legs and abdomen, tenderness of the breasts, weight gain and skin changes. Why women should lack energy at this time is still unknown, but it is almost certainly connected to hormonal effects, possibly a lowering of progesterone levels.

One of the first descriptions of PMS was made in 1937 by Drs McCance, Love and Widdowson in London who reported in the *Journal of Hygiene* on physical and

DID YOU KNOW?

There have been several court cases that have cited PMS as the cause for the defendant's behaviour. They have had varying degrees of success in mitigating the case, although no one has yet been acquitted on the grounds of PMS.

ENERGY BOOST

Ask a friend round for dinner and prepare one of your favourite dishes. Having a good chat over dinner is an excellent way to relieve pressure and unwind.

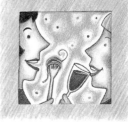

FEMALE REPRODUCTIVE SYSTEM

The main function of the female reproductive system is to provide ova and a safe, comfortable and nutritious environment for their growth and development. The human female is fertile all-year-round, releasing on average an ovum every 28 days. To regulate this complicated system, a number of hormones are produced at different times throughout the cycle, affecting physical and emotional balance.

FEMALE HORMONES
Oestrogen and progesterone prepare the body for pregnancy and peak around ovulation. They are the most important female hormones.

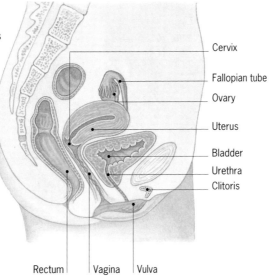

Cervix
Fallopian tube
Ovary
Uterus
Bladder
Urethra
Clitoris

Rectum   Vagina   Vulva

COSMIC ENERGY FORCES: *The Stars*

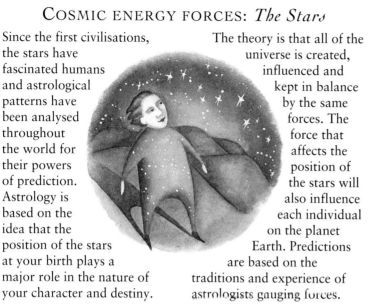

Since the first civilisations, the stars have fascinated humans and astrological patterns have been analysed throughout the world for their powers of prediction. Astrology is based on the idea that the position of the stars at your birth plays a major role in the nature of your character and destiny. The theory is that all of the universe is created, influenced and kept in balance by the same forces. The force that affects the position of the stars will also influence each individual on the planet Earth. Predictions are based on the traditions and experience of astrologists gauging forces.

emotional responses to menstruation. In their detailed study of 167 women they found that fatigue and lack of energy was the most common symptom.

More recently, suggestions have been made that the main cause of premenstrual fatigue is directly related to oestrogen metabolism, in combination with other factors. A number of nutritional imbalances may also occur, including disturbances of iron metabolism and changes in vitamin levels in the body. Supplements of vitamin B_6 and magnesium have been found to help in some cases of PMS, as has taking gamma linolenic acid (GLA), which is a constituent of evening primrose oil and some naturopathic remedies. Try to avoid foods and drinks that contain sugar since premenstrual fatigue is often associated with unstable blood-sugar levels, which are compounded by sporadic intake of sugar.

Although hormone replacement treatment can effectively restore hormonal balance and energy levels and reduce the effects of PMS, it should only be used in extreme cases. The best way to deal with PMS is by organising your life and diet to reduce the symptoms and revitalise your energy as much as possible. One of the first rules is to accept what is happening to your body – much of the fatigue associated with PMS is aggravated by worry that you are unable to do as much as you normally can. Make a note in your diary to remind yourself to avoid stress in the week before your period.

PREGNANCY

The female body undergoes enormous changes during the 40 weeks of pregnancy. The foetus grows progressively and with it conspicuous changes take place in virtually every system of the mother. There is uterine enlargement changing both its shape and function, enlargement of the breasts, increase in blood volume by 30 per cent, and further increases in body weight and respiratory activity. These metabolic

PMS AND MOOD SWINGS

The physical changes involved in the menstrual cycle are well-documented, but the emotional impact of all the hormonal changes is more difficult to gauge. Some of the many research suggestions are shown below.

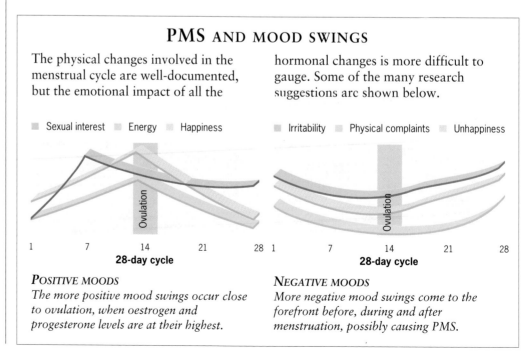

POSITIVE MOODS
The more positive mood swings occur close to ovulation, when oestrogen and progesterone levels are at their highest.

NEGATIVE MOODS
More negative mood swings come to the forefront before, during and after menstruation, possibly causing PMS.

VITAMINS AND MINERALS FOR PREGNANCY

One of the easiest ways to ensure that your pregnancy is healthy and normal is to obtain all the right nutrients in your diet. Doctors advise women to take folic acid supplements prior to pregnancy and during the first 12 weeks.

NUTRIENT	USES	SOURCES
Protein	Provides essential energy for growth	Meat, fish, dairy products, pulses, nuts
Calcium	Forms the building blocks for bones and tissue	Dairy products, sardines, nuts
Vitamin C	Provides material for bones, fights infections	Citrus fruits, berries, green vegetables
Iron	Transfers and transports oxygen	Red meat, fish, egg yolk, green leafy vegetables
Vitamin A	Promotes cell growth and development	Dairy products, eggs, fish, fruit, vegetables
Vitamins B_1, B_2, B_3 and B_6	Metabolise carbohydrate	Wholegrain products
Folic acid	Builds central nervous system	Whole grains, spinach, broccoli, bananas
Vitamin D	Promotes absorption of calcium and phosphorus	Oily fish, eggs, dairy products
Vitamin E	Antioxidant, deficiency can lead to miscarriage	Wheat germ, eggs, sardines, nuts
Phosphorus	Energy metabolism and calcium absorption	Meat, fish, eggs, dairy products, pulses, nuts

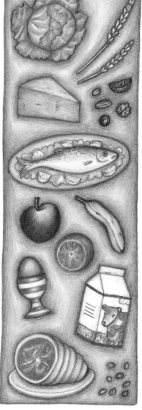

changes, and those of the growing foetus within the mother, demand changes in nutrition and lifestyle. Biologically, the requirements of the foetus are met at the expense of the mother. For example, if the mother does not take sufficient calcium this will be mobilised from her bones to make sure that calcification of the foetal bones occurs correctly.

These physical changes make enormous demands on the diet and lifestyle of the mother, and if due care and attention is not taken the mother could find herself fatigued and lacking in energy.

Dietary balance is essential, with an emphasis on nutrients and vitamins. This ensures that the foetus develops normally and that the mother remains healthy and active. The energy of a pregnant woman is dramatically affected by drugs such as alcohol, nicotine and most medicines, and these should be avoided. Also, hot baths and saunas can cause a rapid increase in body temperature and may be detrimental to the mother's energy levels.

Keeping fit during pregnancy is of great importance and, although excessive energy expenditure and stress on the joints should be avoided, moderate exercise continued throughout pregnancy will be beneficial. The improved energy metabolism, and aerobic and muscular fitness resulting from regular exercise should lead to easier labour and quicker postnatal recovery.

continued on page 34

BIRTHING POSITIONS

The traditional position for giving birth is a sitting or squatting position in which the woman can focus her energy into pushing, and also make use of the force of gravity. It is the preferred position for over 80 per cent of all cultures around the world. It was the usual method of childbirth in Britain until about 200 years ago when 18th-century physicians began to use new techniques, such as forceps, which demanded that the woman lie flat on her back. However, today women have begun to take back control over both position and pain management while giving birth.

FOODS TO AVOID DURING PREGNANCY

Food poisoning from toxoplasmosis or listeriosis can lead to miscarriage or impaired development of the foetus. Foods to avoid include:

▶ *Raw or improperly cooked meats (particularly poultry).*

▶ *Offal, especially liver, may oversupply vitamin A.*

▶ *Soft cheeses.*

▶ *Raw eggs.*

▶ *Some types of raw fish.*

Pregnancy

The nine-month span of pregnancy takes a woman through a variety of physical and emotional phases. Energy levels rise and fall with the demands of foetal growth and as the woman's hormones change. Rest, exercise and a healthy diet are essential.

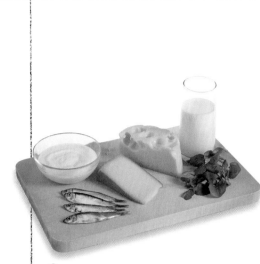

CALCIUM IN THE DIET
Ensure that you are eating enough calcium, as this is necessary for the growth of the baby. High levels are found in milk, yoghurt, cheese, oily fish such as sardines, watercress and other green leafy vegetables.

Understanding the changes that your body is going through is one of the keys to energising your pregnancy. You now have two people to look after through your diet and eating habits, exercise and other health matters. Rest plays an important part in giving your baby the time and energy it needs to develop normally, and you must take every opportunity to relax and take it easy. Biologically the demands of your baby will be met at your own expense, so if you feel tired it may be that your resources have been drained. Making sure that you are eating properly is one of the keys to a successful pregnancy; more information about the nutrients that you need can be found in Chapter 4.

When you feel tired and lacking in energy, it may well be that your body is telling you to rest. Making time to take it easy and avoiding stressful situations can help you to retain high energy levels and encourage the good, healthy growth of your baby. The relaxation techniques on pages 112–13 may enhance your sense of peace and calmness. Exercise also plays a role in good health care and a good balance of rest and exercise is the best strategy (see pages 115–16).

TRIMESTER 1: 0–12 WEEKS

During the first trimester the body is adjusting to your new condition and some of the major hormonal upheavals can be felt towards the end of this period. The metabolic rate rises by between 10–25 per cent due to the energy needed for the baby's growth and for the changes in your own body. This means that you may find your appetite growing and you may quickly become tired or exhausted as all your energy is being focused on the pregnancy.

Your blood pressure is lower during pregnancy and you are more likely to feel faint. A regular food intake and sitting down when you feel tired are the best precautions. Morning sickness may also be a problem in the first trimester. There are no hard and fast remedies for this, except to avoid certain foods that you may feel disagree with you, and rest whenever you feel the need.

▶ *Increase intake of complex carbohydrates*

▶ *Increase intake of fluids*

▶ *Cut out alcohol, caffeine and nicotine*

▶ *Eat little and often, particularly if you are suffering from morning sickness*

▶ *Top up on glucose if you are vomiting*

▶ *Wear a good, supportive bra to help tenderness in the breasts*

DRINKING MORE FLUIDS
Keeping a bottle of mineral water or fruit juice in your bag, so that you can take a sip whenever you need to, is a good way of regularly topping up your fluid intake. Juices contain many of the nutrients needed for pregnancy, are easy to prepare and can be filling.

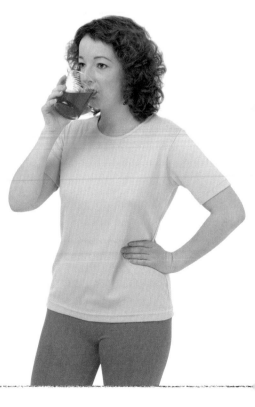

TRIMESTER 2: 13–28 WEEKS

This is the period when you start to feel comfortable with being pregnant. The major hormonal changes will have settled down and hormones are produced in the placenta, rather than the ovaries. The metabolic rate remains high as this is the trimester in which you will gain the most weight and it is essential that you eat well. A rise in progesterone levels may lead to a change in bowel movements which can lead to constipation and other digestive complaints.

▶ *Help to prevent backache with good posture*

▶ *Drink lots of fluids and fibre to help constipation, piles and diarrhoea*

▶ *Keep meals small to deal with longer digestion and heartburn problems*

▶ *Take time to relax*

STANDING POSTURE
It is easy to slip into a bad posture to compensate for the extra weight in front when you are pregnant. Bad posture can lead to backache and prevent ease of movement.

Shoulders should be held square

Bottom should be tucked in

Knees should be slightly bent

Feet should be shoulder-width apart

LIFTING POSTURE
When lifting, bend your knees and use your legs – not your back and shoulders – to lift the object.

Use both hands to lift heavy objects

TRIMESTER 3: 29 WEEKS–DELIVERY

During the third trimester you may well be feeling tired but finding it hard to rest or sleep. Breathing becomes faster and shallower because of the restricted diaphragm movement. This is associated with an increase in carbon dioxide loss, which can make you breathless and lacking in energy. The diaphragm will be relieved when the baby engages in the pelvis in the latest stage of pregnancy, and this will allow you to breathe more easily.

▶ *It may be difficult to sleep for long periods so take naps during the day*

▶ *Try to resist urges to clean and decorate – you'll need your energy for childbirth*

▶ *Relieve water retention problems by sitting down regularly and putting your feet up to help circulation*

▶ *Relieve discomfort in your chest by propping yourself up with cushions*

▶ *Increase fluid and fruit and vegetable intake*

RESTING POSITIONS
The best lying positions are either on your side or on your back. Do not lie flat on your back, however, as this may lead to blood flow problems around your pelvis and abdomen. Cushions and pillows are always handy for making you feel more comfortable.

Raise your top knee with a cushion or pillow

FOOD CRAVINGS

Pregnant women often crave a range of foods, some of which they would not normally favour. Bananas, pickles and ice cream are particularly common examples. The phenomenon is believed to be due to hormone changes unbalancing the system, although it can sometimes also be due to the body demanding nutritional requirements. It is mostly harmless to give in to cravings, especially if the foods are nutritionally wholesome, although you should not eat too many fatty foods. A very rare condition known as pica occurs when pregnant women have a curious desire for non-food substances such as coal, dirt and plaster. This is a more serious problem and you should see a doctor if you find yourself wanting non-foods.

ENDOMETRIOSIS

Endometriosis occurs when the endometrial tissue that lines the uterus is found in other areas of the pelvis. A number of symptoms can be experienced, although pain in the pelvic area, tiredness and fatigue are the most common. It occurs usually between the ages of 30 to 40 and is relatively common: it is found in 20 per cent of gynaecological operations in women of this age. The pain in the pelvis, often at its worst around menstruation, can cause lower back pain and sciatica. It can make sexual intercourse and defecation painful. In severe cases it can interfere with fertility and cause ovarian dysfunction: it is estimated that between 30 and 40 per cent of endometriosis cases result in some degree of infertility.

THE MENOPAUSE

The menopause typically occurs in women around the age of 50, although it can occur at any time from 40 to 60, and occasionally as early as 28. There is usually a period of around two years from the time of the first symptoms until the final cessation of menstruation. A variety of symptoms and effects characterise this period including hot flushes and depression. Along with other hormonal changes that occur with age, there is a reduction in the levels of reproductive hormones, particularly oestrogen – the hormone that is produced primarily in the ovaries. Since the onset of menopause occurs around 50 years of age and women on average now live close to 80 years, it is important that energy disturbances due to hormonal and other changes be rectified.

Many menopausal women complain of lack of energy. This can be overcome with hormonal replacement therapy, although there are alternative methods which are considered more natural and healthy ways of dealing with the problems associated with the menopause.

CAUSES OF CANDIDA OR THRUSH

A thrush infection can grow and infect the vaginal area when the body's defences are lowered. This can be caused by:

▶ *A course of antibiotics killing the body's natural protective bacteria.*

▶ *Hormonal changes due to pregnancy, taking the contraceptive pill or steroids, for example.*

▶ *Restricted air ventilation due to tight or nylon clothing.*

▶ *Hot, damp weather leading to conditions that encourage fungal growth.*

COMMON CAUSES OF FATIGUE

Candida or thrush can have a significant effect on energy levels. It can be treated by applying natural yoghurt to the area. Cystitis is another common problem, sometimes known as the 'honeymoon disease'. It is caused mainly by an infection, often from the large intestine, spreading up the urethra.

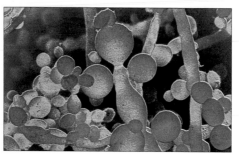

CANDIDA
This electromicrograph depicts the tiny growth of cells that cause the irritation and discomfort of candida or thrush.

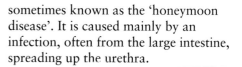

CYSTITIS
This electromicrograph shows the bladder lining ruptured by bacteria (green) causing red blood cells to escape into the urine.

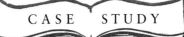
The Fatigued Solicitor

Endometriosis causes pain, a loss of energy, and considerable anxiety both before and during treatment. Understanding the stress factors that often advance the condition may enable the sufferer to resolve problems and alter her lifestyle, improving health and happiness and helping her to fulfil her personal goals.

Esther is 32 years old and makes a good, though stressful, living as a solicitor. She was looking forward to becoming pregnant, with the prospect of being a working mother, until she developed a pain in her lower abdomen about six months ago. It soon became a dragging, incapacitating pain that began four days before her period and lasted until three days after her period had finished. Sex with her husband, Mark, has become painful and the condition has interfered greatly with her work, affecting her concentration and energy levels. She is also finding it difficult to become pregnant and this is causing her further anxiety. Fearing a serious problem with her reproductive system, she visits her doctor.

WHAT SHOULD ESTHER DO?

The cause of the problem needs to be investigated thoroughly and Esther's doctor needs to make a series of tests and examinations, including a full pelvic examination. Having excluded other possible causes, the doctor may use a course of drugs to block menstruation for a couple of months. If the pain stops this clearly links the condition to a reproductive disorder, possibly endometriosis. Esther might then be required to take hormonal preparations to remedy the condition, although surgery may be needed to remove the tissue if the condition persists. Esther would then need to prevent relapse with diet and exercise methods, and use counselling to identify any worries.

STRESS
A stressful job can create a vicious circle of negative influences on your life.

EMOTIONAL HEALTH
Ignoring or avoiding emotional problems can take its toll on your energy.

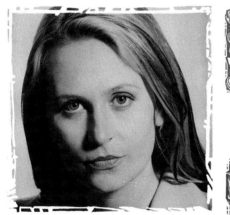

LIFESTYLE
Trying to fit too much into your life can cause health problems.

Action Plan

STRESS
Carefully control stress levels at work and in other areas of life and practise relaxation techniques.

EMOTIONAL HEALTH
Take time to consider emotional problems and work through them properly. Learn to read the signs of growing problems.

LIFESTYLE
Prioritise time and focus on the important parts of life. Do not try to do too much at once. Improve relaxation periods.

HOW THINGS TURNED OUT FOR ESTHER

Esther was diagnosed with endometriosis and needed surgery to remove abnormal endometrial tissue. The health clinic provided her with a diet and exercise routine to prevent the condition from recurring, and counselling helped her to realise that she had been stressed by the prospect of being a working mother. She and Mark decided to cut costs in other areas so that she could relax and stay at home after having the baby.

MEN AND ENERGY

Although men do not undergo the complex hormonal changes that women experience, their energy levels are known to fluctuate enormously due to testosterone production and age.

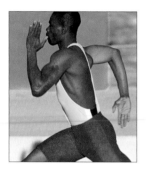

TESTOSTERONE
The hormone that motivates action, drive and performance, testosterone can also contribute to aggression.

In general, men have a higher metabolic rate than women, with higher energy levels, although usually less energy reserved as fats. This is because men have greater amounts of striated muscle and less fat on their bodies. The major fluctuations in male energy levels occur during puberty, when the testes begin to produce the hormone testosterone; as men age, when testosterone levels decrease; and as a result of the effects of alcohol and drugs.

TESTOSTERONE

Testosterone, produced in the testes, is the hormone that stimulates the development of the male primary sexual characteristics and is responsible for the spurt in growth that accompanies puberty. During puberty the dietary needs of a boy rise as he gains height and weight and as his sexual organs mature. The energy value of food becomes increasingly important; boys of this age commonly suffer from fatigue due to poor nutrition, and ensuring that they eat a diet high in protein, carbohydrate and essential nutrients is absolutely crucial.

Testosterone has long been considered the energy hormone for its role in encouraging activity, drive and aggression in men. This hormone has an anabolic, or restorative, effect on body tissues, especially bone marrow and skeletal muscles. This means that if testosterone levels alter, a man may suffer from loss of energy and fatigue, although testosterone can be replaced in the long term by other male hormones produced in the adrenal glands.

Testosterone levels begin to decline after men reach the age of 50, while oestrogen has a tendency to increase. This leads to a general loss of energy, activity and aggression with increasing age. Impotence cannot be redressed with testosterone replacement treatments, although certain fertility disorders can be improved.

Testosterone and illness
Testosterone levels are known to drop away during a variety of illnesses including kidney diseases and liver cirrhosis, and also after stress, surgery, infection or head injury. Low testosterone production may be caused by high alcohol intake or certain drugs, leading to testicular atrophy, or to hormonal changes with age. There are possible benefits of testosterone replacement, although treatments have not been formalised and, to an extent, remain controversial. Low testosterone levels may be found in patients with non-specific illness and poor energy, although the reasons are poorly understood and it is almost certainly a secondary phenomenon.

MALE REPRODUCTIVE SYSTEM

The male reproductive system centres on the testicles and penis. The former produce the male gamete, or sperm, and the hormone testosterone, which develops male characteristics. The penis is used to place the sperm within the reproductive tract of the female for the fertilisation of her ovum.

PROSTATE GLAND
This gland is responsible for releasing lubricating fluids into the urethra. It grows as a result of the hormone changes associated with ageing.

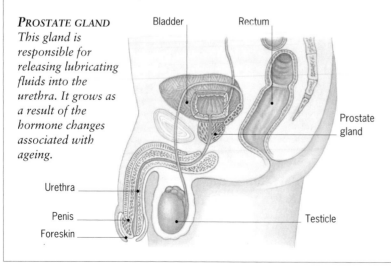

Bladder

Rectum

Prostate gland

Urethra

Penis

Foreskin

Testicle

Impotence

About 10 per cent of all men suffer from impotence, most cases arising after the age of 40 when the body slows down with age. Keeping the body fit and healthy is one of the best measures to counter impotence, enabling you to enjoy a normal sex life.

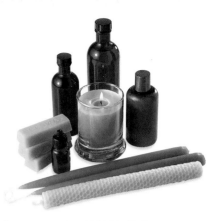

APHRODISIAC MASSAGE OILS
Certain aromatherapy oils have been found to raise libido and levels of sexual stimulation. Mix 5 drops of patchouli, jasmine, rose, sandalwood or ylang ylang essential oil with 25 ml of massage oil. This should be enough for a full, soothing body massage.

Impotence is defined as the inability to get or sustain an erection sufficient for sexual intercourse 75 per cent of the time. Most men experience a weakening of their erection as they grow older, and become progressively less able to perform sex in the usual way. Impotence can also occur if you drink too much alcohol or have too much stress in your life, although it often arises from a combination of factors. Psychological reasons are thought to be the most common underlying reason for impotence, often deriving from stress, anxiety or depression. The best way, therefore, to treat impotence is with relaxation.

THE BENEFITS OF RELAXATION

Relaxation is known to play an important role in learning to live with impotence. Taking the pressure off your own performance and concentrating on pleasing your partner can be a successful method for relaxing you and allowing your body to react naturally.

▶ *Talking over the issue with your partner so that she can understand your problems can help her to help you.*

▶ *Relaxing and taking the time to address the problem and work with it is a crucial element.*

▶ *Aromatherapy massage oils may help relaxation, as can mood music and other aphrodisiacs.*

Aphrodisiacs, such as oysters and shellfish, provide important minerals

Relaxation is the key to tackling impotence problems

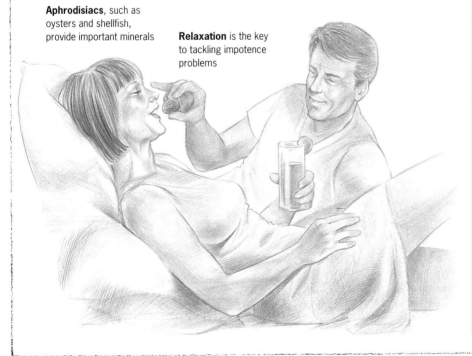

LIFESTYLE TIPS

A healthier lifestyle can help your sex life. Researchers have found the following links:

▶ *Alcohol is a depressant which slows down the body's responses to stimulants, limiting a man's ability to get an erection. It also decreases testosterone production which is linked to lowered libido.*

▶ *A medic in the United States has found that on average if an overweight man loses 35 lbs he will regain an inch of his erection.*

▶ *A fitter lifestyle makes you more able to enjoy sex according to a research study in California.*

▶ *Fat slows the blood and contributes to blockages in the arteries. Maintaining a low-fat diet helps blood to get around your body and penis more efficiently.*

▶ *Smoking is a major factor in impotence, causing blockages in the arteries that prevent blood from entering the penis.*

▶ *Damage to the penis can be a cause of impotence, although this is less common.*

ENERGY BOOST

Bringing a piece of nature inside can add natural energy to a room, and should last for a week or more. If it is winter, a few twigs and branches, perhaps with pine or fir cones, can enliven the atmosphere. According to Norse and Saxon mythology, the logs and branches brought in at Christmas come from the idea of the Tree of Life, which is said to support the Earth, heaven and hell. You can combine them in a display with evergreen sprigs, such as holly, a fertility and life-bringing tradition from ancient Mesopotamia.

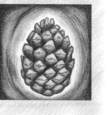

Both athletes and non-athletes have tried to boost their energy levels with doses of testosterone, although without any effect. It has, however, been found that testosterone supplements can cause major medical problems, such as liver damage, apart from when they are used to replace impaired production of the hormone.

PROSTATE PROBLEMS

The prostate is a small, chestnut-sized gland at the base of the bladder and surrounding the top part of the urethra. It is responsible for secretions that keep the urethra moist and the production of the seminal fluids released during ejaculation. The position of the prostate under the bladder means that any problems it incurs can cause discomfort to the bladder and the urinary system.

By far the most common problem is an enlarged prostate, which occurs in most men over the age of 50. Other less common conditions include cancer of the prostate, and prostatitis – a bacterial infection – both of which must be treated by a doctor.

FOODS RICH IN ZINC AND VITAMIN B6
Many men find relief from prostate trouble by eating a diet rich in zinc and vitamin B6. Zinc can be found in shellfish, nuts and seeds, red meat and whole grains. Vitamin B6 is available from bananas, vegetables, whole grains, liver and nuts.

Enlarged prostate

An enlarged prostate, also known as benign prostatic hypertrophy, occurs as the body's hormones change with age and results in pressure on the bladder and the need to urinate frequently. It is not known exactly what causes the problem, although it has been suggested that it is linked with the depletion of testosterone and the increase in other hormones, such as oestrogen, which can occur at any time after the age of 40. As the prostate grows it obstructs the passage of urine from the bladder, leaving the sufferer needing to urinate frequently, often during the night. This can severely disrupt sleep patterns and lead to tiredness and fatigue through the day. The condition can eventually cause chronic outflow obstruction, leading to a deterioration of kidney function and an increase of urea in the bloodstream, which can ultimately result in serious medical problems.

The hormone prolactin is believed to antagonise the situation further by encouraging more testosterone to be taken up by the prostate and to increase the synthesis of dihydrotestosterone. Since prolactin levels are increased by beer and stress, these factors contribute greatly to an enlarged prostate and should be avoided. Drugs can be taken to reduce prolactin levels, although these are known to have side effects. Some doctors and practitioners recommend a diet high in both zinc and vitamin B6 which can reduce prolactin levels in a more natural way (see page 100).

DID YOU KNOW?

Men can stay fertile well into their old age. The oldest known father in Britain was Frank Tawney of Somerset who was 93 years old when his wife, Elizabeth, who was 50 years younger than him, gave birth to a baby boy on 21 January 1987.

CHAPTER 2

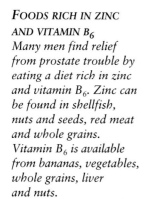

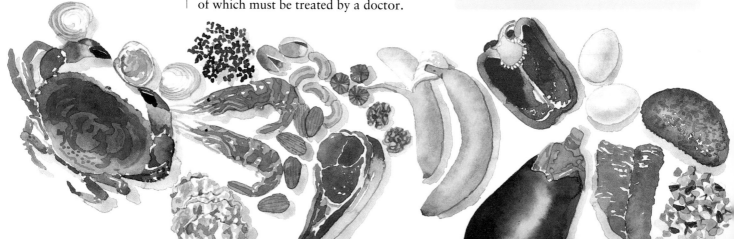

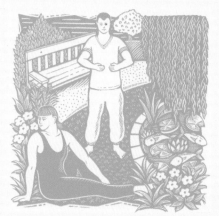

THE ENERGY ALL AROUND US

We are constantly bombarded by energy, both from natural sources, such as the sun and the elements, and from man-made sources, such as electricity carried by overhead power lines. These forces can affect us for both good and bad, and many have been harnessed by orthodox and complementary medicine to improve our energy levels and all-round health.

LIGHT AND COLOUR

Perhaps the most powerful form of energy that affects our lives is light, with the associated forces of colour and heat. These energies are used in both conventional and alternative health.

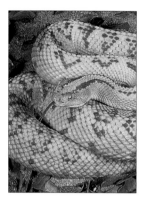

ANIMAL INSIGHT
Many creatures are aware of energy wavelengths other than those that humans can sense. Insects such as bees and butterflies see UV light, while rattlesnakes detect specific infrared waves through their skin.

Light, colour and heat energy are all forms of electromagnetic radiation and are utilised in both conventional medicine, for example in the form of x-rays and radiotherapy, and complementary therapies, such as in light therapy.

LIGHT AND COLOUR

We are only consciously aware of a narrow band of wavelengths in the middle of the electromagnetic spectrum. We can see light (the visible spectrum) and we can feel heat (infrared waves) and our skins are tanned by ultraviolet light. We cannot sense wavelengths above and below this, although they can be detected by technical instruments and may often affect our bodies and health in subtle ways.

Different wavelengths of visible light are seen as different colours – violet, indigo, blue, green, yellow, orange and red. These are the rainbow colours that make up the visible spectrum. When white light falls on an object some wavelengths are absorbed while others are reflected. If, for example, only the wavelength that makes blue light is reflected we will see the object as blue. If all wavelengths of light are reflected we see the object as white. If all the wavelengths are absorbed, however, we see it as black.

LIGHT IN MEDICINE

Various wavelengths of light are employed in conventional medicine. Treatment with light is called phototherapy and includes the use of visible light, UV light and concentrated light beams known as lasers.

Visible light is used to treat a form of winter depression called seasonal affective disorder (SAD). This condition mainly affects people living in northerly latitudes during the winter when daylight is limited. Sunlight and UV light, often in combination with drugs, are used to treat skin disorders such

THE ELECTROMAGNETIC SPECTRUM

All objects emit heat radiation, which consists of electromagnetic waves. These waves, collectively known as the electromagnetic spectrum, radiate at different wavelengths, some narrow and concentrated, such as x-rays and gamma rays, and others wide and less powerful, such as radio waves. The sun is the most powerful source of electromagnetic radiation. It sends out all forms of radiation – not just light and heat. All electromagnetic radiation travels at the speed of light and passes easily through space.

ELECTROMAGNETIC WAVELENGTH
Each group of waves has a different wavelength and carries a different amount of energy. For example, radio waves have a longer wavelength and less energy than short-wave x-rays.

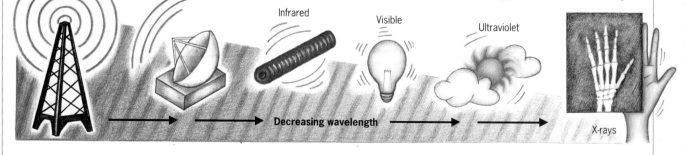

Radio

Microwaves

Infrared

Visible

Ultraviolet

Decreasing wavelength

X-rays

Colour Therapy

Colour has a powerful effect on your mood. It can be used to enhance or change your emotions and reduce negative thoughts by encouraging positive ones to dominate. Colour therapies can be used to channel your energy in positive directions.

Colour therapy is a system of complementary treatment which harnesses the radiant energy that emanates from the light-giving properties of different colours. Although it has no scientific backing, we are all aware of our reactions to colour, and the therapy attributes specific colours to various parts of the body and to specific disorders.

Colour therapists work in many different ways, such as through fixing a concentrated beam of coloured light over a troubled area of the body. Blue babies have been successfully treated with yellow lights in this way. Many other alternative therapies, such as Ayurvedic medicine, use colour to enhance other treatments.

FINDING YOUR COLOURS
Close your eyes and visualise your energising colours. Imagine yourself in a room of each colour and how you respond. Choose the colour that best suits your personal energies.

USING COLOURS TO BRIGHTEN YOUR LIFE

If you want to change a negative way of thinking into a more positive one, choose a colour from the list below with attributes you would like to encourage within yourself. Wear that colour throughout the day, or have objects surrounding you with that colour, and positive thoughts will occur to you whenever you look at the colour. It may sound simplistic, but carefully colouring your clothes and environment can help you to balance the forces within you, increasing your energy and making you feel more positive.

COLOUR ALL AROUND YOU
To improve your energy, redecorate a room in your home in a colour you feel inspires energy. Alternatively, you can use the colour in soft furnishings, clothes and accessories.

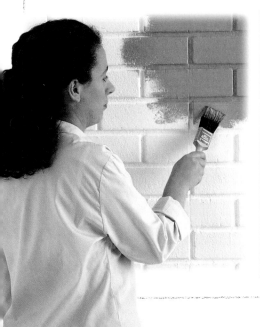

EMOTIONAL EFFECTS

Colour therapists use eight main colours to encourage certain emotions and attitudes, usually by surrounding the patient with that colour. White is considered to have cleansing properties.

COLOUR	ATTRIBUTES
Red	Energising, strengthening, promotes vitality. Helps overcome fatigue and inertia
Orange	Happiness, joy, carefree, uplifting to the spirit. Helps to treat depression and low energy levels
Yellow	Promotes intellectual thought and clear thinking. Improves judgment
Green	Helps to achieve harmony and balance. Cleanses and purifies the spirit
Turquoise	Promotes calmness and strengthens immunity. Helps overcome nervous tension
Blue	Induces calm and relaxation. Promotes feelings of peacefulness
Violet	Spiritually uplifting. Improves self-respect and esteem. Provides hope
Magenta	Encourages the breaking of habits and letting go of old emotions. Promotes sense of freedom and release

COSMIC ENERGY FORCES: *Thunder*

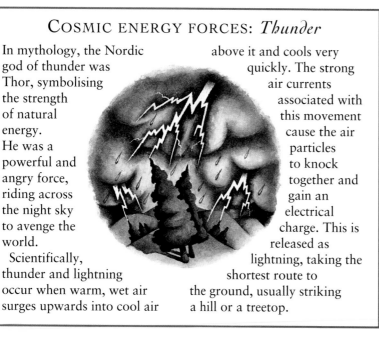

In mythology, the Nordic god of thunder was Thor, symbolising the strength of natural energy. He was a powerful and angry force, riding across the night sky to avenge the world.

Scientifically, thunder and lightning occur when warm, wet air surges upwards into cool air above it and cools very quickly. The strong air currents associated with this movement cause the air particles to knock together and gain an electrical charge. This is released as lightning, taking the shortest route to the ground, usually striking a hill or a treetop.

PROTECTING YOUR SKIN FROM THE SUN

Protection against the UV rays of the sun helps to prevent burning, sunstroke and skin cancer, and is especially important for people with fair skin. There are many ways to protect yourself against UV rays.

▶ *Use protective cream or sunblock on your skin.*

▶ *Wear a wide-brimmed hat which shades your face to protect your facial skin. A hat will also protect against sunstroke.*

▶ *Stay in the shade, or move to the shade after every half hour in the sunshine.*

▶ *Wear light clothes that cover your skin.*

---

as vitiligo and psoriasis. Visible blue light is employed to treat a form of jaundice that affects newborn babies.

Low-intensity lasers are used to treat damaged muscles, ligaments, tendons and joints. The laser generates heat which reduces inflammation and pain, improves the flow of blood and lymph, and stimulates tissue healing. High-intensity lasers can be used to cut away scar tissue, remove abnormal cells and cancer growths, seal damaged blood vessels and also to break up kidney and gallstones.

You are mainly aware of UV light through its action on your skin. UV rays activate cells in the skin to increase production of the pigment melanin, which causes the characteristic darkening familiar as a sun tan. Overexposure to UV light causes burning and skin damage.

Colour therapy

Colours have long been known to have a powerful influence on mood. Those at the lower end of the visible spectrum, such as violet and blue, are considered restful and thoughtful; they are associated with peace and study, and believed to be beneficial for stress and anxiety. Those at the higher end of the spectrum, such as red, orange and yellow, are vibrant, energetic colours associated with elation, activity and passion.

Colour therapy employs different colours for their mood-enhancing properties and for other therapeutic qualities they are thought to possess. For example, surrounding yourself with energetic colours, through redecorating your walls or wearing those colours, counteracts depression. Special concentrated lights can also be employed to counter specific problems.

X-RAY RADIATION

One of the most common forms of energy used in medical diagnosis, x-ray radiation enables photographs to be taken of bones and internal organs. X-rays were discovered in 1895 by the German physicist Wilhelm Roentgen. They are part of the electromagnetic spectrum, to which ultraviolet (UV) light, visible light, infrared and radio waves also belong.

X-rays tend to pass through softer tissues but are easily absorbed by denser tissue and bone. Although invisible to the human eye, x-rays darken photographic film. Because of this, x-ray cameras have been used for almost a century to photograph bones to check for possible fractures. The stomach or intestines can be visualised after consuming a barium meal – barium is impervious to x-rays and so outlines the organ, showing up problem areas.

Early forms of x-ray cameras used high levels of radiation that caused a greatly increased risk of cancer. Modern methods use very low levels, especially computed tomography (CT) scanning and positron emission tomography (PET) which produce three-dimensional computer images.

Radiotherapy

Since the turn of the century, x-rays and other forms of radiation have been used to cure disorders as well as to diagnose them. This form of treatment, called radiotherapy, involves directing the x-rays at unwanted cells such as cancer cells to destroy them. Early forms of radiotherapy also tended to damage neighbouring healthy tissue, but modern systems are more accurate and direct the radiation only onto the tumour. Instead of x-rays, some forms of radiotherapy involve neutron beams, and substances such as radioactive iodine and yttrium.

Radiotherapy is often combined with surgery and chemotherapy, or drug therapy, to treat cancers of the breast, larynx, skin, cervix, oesophagus and blood (leukaemia). It can also be used on other conditions, such as an overactive thyroid.

THE POWER OF MAGNETISM

There is much scientific debate about the possible therapeutic effects of magnetism. It is known that an electrically generated form of magnetism, called electromagnetism, plays a part in living processes, particularly nerve and muscle activity, brain function and metabolism. In every cell, there are estimated to be 100 000 interactions per second involving electromagnetism at a molecular level. Magnetism is found naturally in metals, is detectable in the Earth's magnetic field, or can be produced electronically. Studies on US astronauts conducted by the National Aeronautics and Space Administration (NASA) in the 1960s discovered that many were suffering from a form of space sickness caused by living for extended periods outside the Earth's magnetic field, known as the magnetosphere. This had a serious effect on the circulation and oxygenation of their blood and was only corrected by fitting magnets to the space craft.

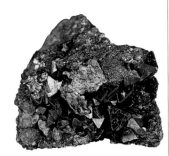

THE EARTH'S MAGNETIC FIELD
The magnetic force of the Earth has a major influence on our lives. The physical functioning of astronauts is disrupted if they remain in space for extended periods.

Magnets have been used for many centuries to ease inflammatory joint disorders, such as arthritis. In the late 1950s, two doctors, Robert Becker and Andrew Bassett, used electromagnetic fields to treat patients with gangrene in their leg tissue. Electromagnetism proved effective in aiding tissue repair in cases where the limb would otherwise have been at risk. Despite their success, however, the therapeutic uses of magnetism are mostly confined to complementary health.

Magnet therapy is based on the belief that physical disorders are mainly due to imbalances in the electromagnetic fields generated by the body's cells. Placing magnets over the problem area is believed to have a rebalancing effect on the body and so alleviate the disorder.

Magnetic rocks known as bloodstones have been mined in Africa for thousands of years and added to medicinal potions or placed on the skin to treat disease. The ancient Greeks and Chinese used the healing properties of magnetic rocks called lodestones.

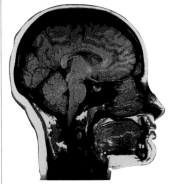

Magnetic resonance imaging (MRI) is a diagnostic technique using magnetism to build up images of the internal organs. The patient lies inside a very large electromagnet which causes atoms in the tissues to align. The atoms are then knocked out of alignment with pulses of radio waves, causing them to broadcast radio signals which can be used to build up an image. MRI can be used to examine the brain, spinal cord, heart, blood vessels, bones and endocrine glands. It is a technique complementary to x-ray imaging.

Magnetising water for drinking or bathing is a traditional Indian therapy. Water can be magnetised by placing the opposite poles of two magnets on each side of a glass of water for 12–18 hours. The water should be used fairly quickly following the treatment, and must not be refrigerated. The water is believed to improve health by balancing the energy forces within each cell through which it promotes vitality and strength, especially in the organs.

Electromagnetic field therapy (EMF) is a modern form of magnet therapy that is widely used in Eastern and Central Europe, but is less commonly used in either Western Europe or North America. It involves the use of small portable generators which produce low-frequency pulsating electromagnetic fields in order to rebalance the body. It is claimed to treat a wide range of disorders including arthritis, nerve disorders, fractures and urinary complaints.

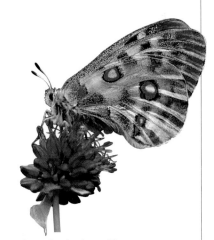

Magnetic navigation is used by many creatures to locate themselves. Animals such as homing pigeons and emperor butterflies can detect the Earth's magnetic field and use it to navigate vast distances.

SOUND

Everybody has experienced the uplifting effects of sound through music and song, and the therapeutic use of sound in health care is now starting to become more widespread.

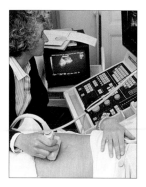

ULTRASOUND
The most common use for ultrasound imaging is to view the foetus of an unborn baby in the mother's womb.

MUSIC AND DANCING
Dancing can be energising and uplifting, providing good exercise and making you feel great. A natural form of stress relief, dancing is enjoyed by every culture in the world.

Sound is a series of pressure waves, or 'sound waves', moving through a medium such as air or water. In air, sound waves travel at 332 metres (1089 feet) per second, but are even faster in water, at 1482 metres (4863 feet) per second. When sound waves strike an object they cause it to vibrate, or 'resonate'.

Sound is split into waves of different lengths. If sound waves of the right length strike the eardrum they cause it to resonate, which the brain perceives as 'sound'. Sound frequencies within the range of human hearing are known as sonic. Frequencies below this are called subsonic, and above this are called supersonic, or ultrasonic.

ULTRASOUND

The technique that bats and dolphins use to navigate is called echolocation and is the basic principle behind ultrasound, an imaging technique widely employed in conventional medicine. With ultrasound, high-frequency sound waves are directed at the part of the body to be examined using a device called a transducer. This device also

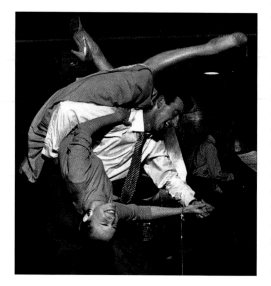

detects the echoes from internal organs and transmits them to a computer, which uses the information to create an image. The technique is commonly used to monitor the development of an unborn baby in utero.

Ultrasound is most effective for examining soft tissues and fluid-filled structures such as the heart, breasts, kidneys, liver, gall bladder, pancreas, ovaries and testes. It is also used in physiotherapy to promote tissue growth and repair, for example, on a torn ligament or muscle strain.

SOUND THERAPY

Throughout recorded history, sound has been used in different ways to treat mental and physical disorders. The simplest use of sound is through singing, chanting and playing or listening to music. Sound employed in this way is known to act as a mood enhancer, to relieve severe mental states such as depression and anxiety, and to reduce chronic stress.

According to Ayurvedic teaching, the world began with a pure, formless 'cosmic consciousness' from which arose a soundless vibration called 'aum'. Aum, or om, is often chanted as a mantra during meditation sessions to help people to tune in to a higher plane of consciousness.

By intoning sounds of specific frequencies, practitioners aim to target one of seven energy centres or 'chakras' located along a straight line between the base of the spine and the crown of the head. Chakras, from the Sanskrit word for 'wheel', spin faster or slower according to the energy flowing through them. In sound therapy, sound is directed to rebalance the system and open up the energy channels. Sound can either be chanted by others towards the patient, or it may be generated by an electronic device which is set to the correct frequency to treat the specific condition.

Sound Therapy

Ancient cultures have harnessed sound as a means of expressing inner emotions and use its resonance to heal the body and spirit. Sound therapy can greatly help emotional problems, particularly depression and feelings connected with isolation.

Sound therapists believe that the organs and cells of the body react to vibrating sound. According to the principles behind the therapy, the body responds well to a natural resonance which reacts favourably to other sounds that are compatible. Sounds which resonate unfavourably on a particular organ produce discord and disharmony, and can result in ill health. To treat physical or emotional disorders, practitioners direct harmonious or therapeutic sounds at the area of the body believed to be causing the problem.

The underlying theory holds that each part of the body has its own natural resonance and will vibrate in harmony with any sound of the same frequency. The same principle causes a wine glass to resonate when a singer reaches a particular musical note. Disease is thought to dampen down the frequency at which the affected organ or body part vibrates. Sound waves of the correct frequency vibrate the tissues so that they resonate normally again and become stronger and better able to fight the disease.

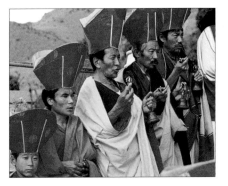

MEDITATIVE CHANTING
Many religions use the power of the human voice to inspire spiritual and emotional well-being. These Buddhist monks are chanting to gain spiritual enlightenment.

Sound is also believed to open the energy channels of the body and is therefore used in a number of Eastern health treatments.

CHANTING TO RELIEVE DEPRESSION

Chanting is an ancient tradition used by many cultures to induce a spiritual, meditative or uplifting mood. In Eastern cultures, chanting is used to increase spiritual awareness and inner tranquillity. In the West, chanting also has its part to play. Most traditional religious ceremonies rely on voice to recite prayers and sing hymns in praise of nature and God, intoning the serious spiritual message of the ceremony.

The traditional Hindu *om* mantra consists of three sounds: aah (which vibrates in your navel), oo (which vibrates in your heart), and m (which vibrates in your temple).

Sit comfortably and ensure that you can breathe easily and properly

1 *Sit somewhere quiet where you can be peaceful. Relax your body so your diaphragm is free to move. Dim the lights in the room if this helps you to concentrate. Clear your mind and breathe deeply for a few moments.*

2 *Quietly at first, chant your words. These could be the words to a song you have always found uplifting or words you have devised yourself. They could take the form of affirmations or prayer. They must be positive and confirming. For example, you could chant: 'every day I become stronger', 'I am at one with the world', or 'love is within and around me'.*

3 *After each chant, take a deep breath before you commence your next chant. Your voice level may rise as you gain confidence.*

ANIMALS, VEGETABLES AND MINERALS

The life energies within the kingdom of nature can be drawn upon to balance your own energies, as can the energy from the mineral elements which form a basis for all life.

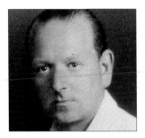

The energy of plants and minerals has been used for thousands of years to promote health and vitality. The ancient Egyptians were particularly keen to take advantage of the natural energies of both plants and minerals, especially precious stones which were mounted in jewellery or in ornaments to preserve positive energies. According to traditional Chinese medicine, natural energies from herbs and stones contribute greatly to energy balance.

The native American Indians wear feathers, particularly of birds of prey, to partake of the birds' natural energies. The skins and furs of animals are also used for this purpose. Once again, it is the skins of powerful animals that are used, so that the wearer can take on the characteristic strength of, say, the bear or the buffalo. Many other cultures around the world, notably the peoples of West Africa, have used teeth and bones from animals for their energising qualities.

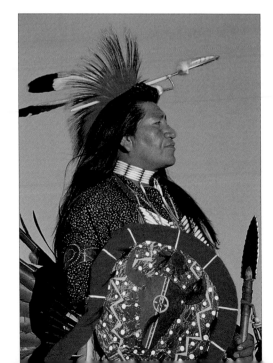

HOMEOPATHY

Homeopathic medicine puts great store by the concept of energy, or 'vital force', that exists in plants, minerals and other natural substances. In homeopathy, the plant material is extracted in a water/ethanol medium. The mixture is shaken in a process called succession which is believed to impart the vital force of the ingredient to the water. The solution is taken orally in small doses.

Homeopathic remedies are based on the principle of 'like cures like': substances which in large doses produce symptoms that mimic a particular disease will, in small amounts, actually cure the illness. The therapy was prompted by the discovery that cinchona bark, from which the antimalarial drug quinine is extracted, itself produces malaria-like symptoms, such as fever.

The active ingredients in homeopathic remedies are so dilute that no trace of the original ingredient can be detected. Yet numerous studies have shown that homeopathic remedies can be highly beneficial in alleviating a wide range of illnesses. Some practitioners believe that this is because the process of succession transfers the ingredient's vital force to the water's molecular structure. However, there are many theories but no clear and coherent explanation of how homeopathy works.

FLOWER REMEDIES

Extracts of flowers and other plants have been used for thousands of years to treat illness, but their active ingredients can also be diluted, like homeopathic remedies, in order to enhance their vital force. The best-known exponent of the healing powers of flowers was Edward Bach, a practising doctor and homeopath in the early 20th century.

Bach devised a simple treatment system based on 38 flower remedies. He believed that the essence of the flower could be extracted by allowing it to float on clear spring water in sunlight for a few hours.

Flower remedies are mainly used for alleviating psychological disorders such as mental trauma, stress and depression. According to Bach, the essences of his flower remedies contain a life force which vibrates at a higher level than mere flesh and blood.

MINERALS

Minerals have been used for many years as sources of decoration, and some have been attributed with special forces. Until the last century, folk doctors applied gold leaf to wounds in order to speed the healing process, although their success was questionable. Other metals attributed with special forces include silver and copper.

CRYSTALS

Due to their precise structure, crystals resonate at a constant rate, which is why quartz crystals are used in watches to keep accurate time. When quartz crystals are put in an electromagnetic field they vibrate at a high frequency, thus producing ultrasonic sounds. This is the principle behind ultrasound scanners. By bouncing these sounds off internal organs in the body they can be used to investigate medical disorders.

Crystal therapy

The precise structures of crystals, often forming into arrangements of cubes or octahedrons (eight-sided figures), has long fascinated alternative therapists. Many believe the stones can contain powerful energy forces. Some therapists argue that they can treat physical, mental, emotional and spiritual ills by correcting imbalances in the vibration patterns in the body's tissues.

Some therapists use crystals on a pendulum to aid diagnosis. A crystal is suspended over the area of the body being investigated, and by its movements the therapist locates the underlying cause. To treat a condition, a crystal may be placed next to the body for a while, or individuals may be told to wear the crystal or carry it around with them. Some people sew small pockets into their inner garments in which to carry crystals.

Crystal-essence therapy involves the use of liquid remedies. These consist of pure water that has been energised through contact with crystals in bright sunlight. The individual places a few drops of the remedy under the tongue at certain times of the day.

Electrocrystal therapy uses electricity to increase the resonance of crystals. The crystals are placed in a saline-filled glass tube and sealed. The tube is then placed on the body and electrically stimulated at a pulse rate that matches the natural resonance of the part of the body being treated.

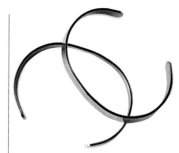

*COPPER BRACELETS FOR ARTHRITIS
Research in Australia in the early 1980s found that the copper in a bracelet can penetrate the skin and act as an anti-inflammatory agent on arthritis and rheumatism.*

THE ENERGY OF STONES

With their regular shapes and smooth surfaces, crystals are created by the strong electromagnetic attraction of one atom to others of the same kind. Some therapists see this as evidence of great energy and healing power. Other semi-precious stones are also associated with particular powers. Crystals may be carried on the person or kept in the home.

*HEALING STONES?
Crystal therapy associates each crystal with a different physical, mental or spiritual attribute, some examples of which are shown here. They may be used individually or in combination.*

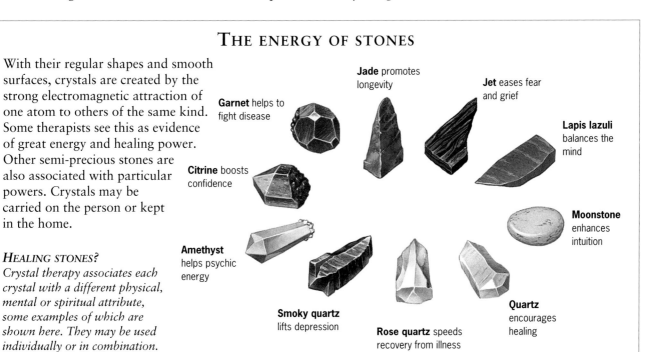

Garnet helps to fight disease

Jade promotes longevity

Jet eases fear and grief

Lapis lazuli balances the mind

Citrine boosts confidence

Moonstone enhances intuition

Amethyst helps psychic energy

Smoky quartz lifts depression

Rose quartz speeds recovery from illness

Quartz encourages healing

THE FIVE ENERGIES

Ayurveda and traditional Chinese medicine share a belief in five principal forces of energy that govern the world around us, as well as our own physical, mental and psychological health.

THE FIVE ELEMENTS AND YOUR BODY

Each of the five elements is connected to a yin and a yang part of the body. If you have an imbalance in your elements, it may manifest itself physically in this region.

► *Wood has the liver as the yin organ and the gall bladder as the yang.*

► *Fire's yin organ is the heart, and yang is the small intestine.*

► *Earth can be found in the spleen (yin) and the stomach (yang).*

► *Metal has the lungs as the yin organ and the large intestine as the yang.*

► *Water's yin organ is the kidney, and the yang is the bladder.*

SEASONS AND ENERGY
According to traditional Chinese medicine, your energy levels are strongly affected by the dominant energy force of the season. For example, spring is characterised by young yang energy and the element wood. This energy force can tend towards excess and aggression, and so some therapists recommend yin foods to achieve balance (see page 75).

Many people are aware of the influence of the seasons and weather patterns on mood and energy level. For some people, a change in humidity or temperature may bring about illness or aggravate an existing condition such as asthma. However, in Ayurveda and traditional Chinese medicine five fundamental energy forces of nature are seen as directing our health and well-being. Good health involves ensuring a proper balance of the five basic energies.

AYURVEDIC MEDICINE
Ayurvedic medicine originated in India over 4000 years ago and is based on an understanding of prana, the natural energy or life force. According to Ayurvedic teaching, nature and all matter – including people – is made up of five elements: earth, water, fire, air and ether (space). In different combinations, these elements make up the three principles, or tridoshas – vata, pita and kapha – that govern all things.

The principle of the three doshas is at the heart of Ayurveda (see page 50). Each is made up of combinations of two of the elements. Vata, which represents winter, com-

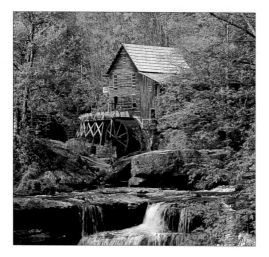

bines ether and air and controls movement. Pita signifies summer and combines fire and water, and is responsible for metabolism. Kapha represents spring and combines water and earth. It is responsible for growth and structure, the solid, unmoving factor.

As people are considered to be a microcosm of the natural world, they too are defined by one or more of the tridoshas and their relevant elements. Ayurvedic treatments aim to balance the tridoshas, bringing a person's elements into harmony and helping them to understand their strengths and weaknesses.

THE FIVE ELEMENT THEORY
The principles of Ayurveda spread to China where they were modified and, over time, developed into the principles of traditional Chinese medicine. The equivalent to prana is chi, which means 'breath' or 'spirit'. It is the life force or vital energy found in all living things, and forms the five elements – fire, air, wood, metal and earth.

Each person should have a balance of the five energies, and if one is dominant or submissive, it should be balanced by using an opposing energy to 'control' or 'nourish' the problem area. Energy problems are investigated and diagnosed by examining the body, mental attitude and emotions. Commonly a patient has a specific problem that needs treatment, such as a stomach problem which would be identified as an earth disorder. The treatment would encourage strength and balance of the earth energy by stifling the 'controlling' force and encouraging the 'nourishing' force.

Practitioners treat imbalances with a combination of remedies including dietary measures, lifestyle changes, herbalism, massage (Tui Na), exercises (chi kung) and acupuncture. A psychological element helps with both diagnosis and treatment, and can also

THE FIVE ELEMENTS

Each person is created from a mixture of the five elements, and a balance of all five energies breeds health and energy. However, people have imbalances which affect their physical and psychological make-up. To redress an imbalance, the problem is identified by matching the symptoms, and the problem element is then controlled or encouraged by observing and treating the other elements through herbal treatments, acupuncture, changes in diet and mental attitude and exercises (see Chapter 5). You can find out your astrological element from the table on page 52.

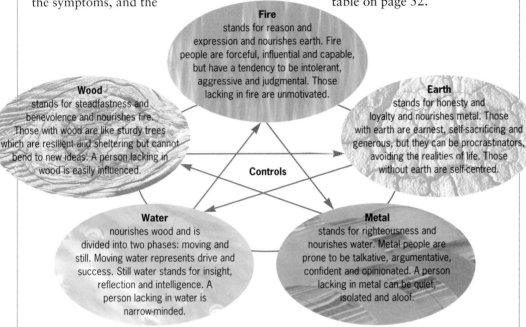

Fire
stands for reason and expression and nourishes earth. Fire people are forceful, influential and capable, but have a tendency to be intolerant, aggressive and judgmental. Those lacking in fire are unmotivated.

Wood
stands for steadfastness and benevolence and nourishes fire. Those with wood are like sturdy trees which are resilient and sheltering but cannot bend to new ideas. A person lacking in wood is easily influenced.

Earth
stands for honesty and loyalty and nourishes metal. Those with earth are earnest, self-sacrificing and generous, but they can be procrastinators, avoiding the realities of life. Those without earth are self-centred.

Controls

Water
nourishes wood and is divided into two phases: moving and still. Moving water represents drive and success. Still water stands for insight, reflection and intelligence. A person lacking in water is narrow-minded.

Metal
stands for righteousness and nourishes water. Metal people are prone to be talkative, argumentative, confident and opinionated. A person lacking in metal can be quiet, isolated and aloof.

How it works

The following example illustrates how the five element theory works in practice. If you have a kidney problem, you may have a water disorder. Since earth controls water, your problem may be due to an overactive soil element, possibly originating in the spleen or stomach. Treat it by nourishing water with metal foods and emotions. You may also need to consider the psychological aspects of the problem: are you anxious about anything? What do you have to fear?

be used for predictions, especially in combination with Chinese astrology. The holistic approach of traditional Chinese medicine stresses the direct link between the body, personality and behaviour. A change in lifestyle and attitude is often equally as important as physical treatments to restore health and vitality.

Traditional Chinese practitioners believe that there are other powerful forces in nature as well as chi and the five elements. The most important of these are yin and yang, which are seen as opposing yet complementary poles, forces or principles. Yin is the cold, passive, feminine force, while yang is the warm, active, masculine force. Yin and yang exist in all things in different proportions but maintain a state of equilibrium unless malign forces upset this balance. An imbalance in yin and yang causes disharmony in nature and physical illness in people, and Chinese medicine is aimed at restoring and maintaining the balance between these two forces.

CHINESE ASTROLOGY AND THE FIVE ELEMENTS

Traditional Chinese philosophy suggests that each year is represented by an animal and an element, and that these will dictate continued on page 52

DID YOU KNOW?

Western astrology and the study of the star signs originated in India and is based on the traditional reading of the stars and planets to perceive the changes and imbalances in universal forces. It is founded on a system of 12 signs dependent on the changing arrangements of stars and planets as the Earth moves throughout the year. Each sign has a ruling element, although Western astrology recognises only four signs: earth, water, air and fire. These affect the personality and health of each individual in a similar fashion to the Ayurvedic elements and the five element theory.

Ayurveda Practitioner

The principle of energy balancing has a central role in Ayurvedic medicine. The therapy takes a holistic approach to ailments and examines how diet, exercise and emotions work together to influence your health and energy levels.

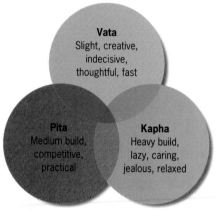

THE TRIDOSHA
Ayurvedic tradition holds that each individual is a mixture of three characters, with different physical, health and emotional natures. If you have a health problem, you are assessed for which dosha is out of balance and this forms the basis of treatment.

Ayurvedic medicine, the traditional and all-encompassing system of Indian medicine, derives its name from the Sanskrit for life (*ayur*) and knowledge (*veda*). The system is holistic, aiming to treat imbalances of mind, body and spirit to promote good health and combat illness. It is widely used in India alongside orthodox medicine and is now gaining interest in the West.

How does Ayurvedic medicine work?
Ayurvedic medicine is an ancient medical practice that is based on the concept of prana (energy). This energy is forever fluctuating, changing from negative to positive and back again, and controls our physical, mental, emotional and spiritual health. The aim of an

Ayurvedic practitioner is to balance or promote more positive energy in all these areas to allow us to achieve our full potential in life.

There are three different types of person in Ayurvedic medicine and each type represents one of the tridoshas – vata, pita and kapha. Most people are combinations of two or all three in varying degrees. Your dominant and combined doshas determine your physical shape, constitution, colouring, personality and temperament, as well as the types of illness you might suffer from. They also determine how you are treated.

What happens during a session?
Ayurvedic practitioners believe strongly in the individual and how that person reacts to the world. For this reason, it is accepted that not all remedies will work in the same way for everyone. The skill of the practitioner is to identify and prescribe treatment that will work for the individual. To achieve this, the practitioner will aim to find out as much about the patient as is possible. This will include medical details about you, your parents and your grandparents, as it is from them that you inherit your body type and constitution. Also, reincarnation and karma (the result of your actions in previous lives) are key Ayurvedic principles, and these are also explored. You will be closely questioned about your diet, lifestyle and sexual behaviour. Finally, your actual symptoms will be investigated.

Origins
Ayurvedic medicine originated in India some 4000 years ago. A group of 52 wise and holy men left their homes and went to the Himalayas, as the mountains were believed to be closer to universal forces. There, they meditated on how they could learn to eradicate illness from the world. Their meditations, which they believed were divinely inspired, led them to devise principles and systems to promote good health. They wrote these down in the *Charaka Samhita*, which is regarded as a sacred text.

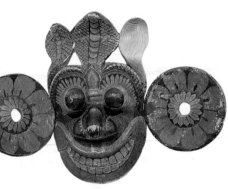

HEALING MASK
Masks are traditionally used to ward off the demons that upset the balance of the tridosha. This mask represents Garayaka, the demon of purification, and is worn to exorcise the evil spirit. It is from Sri Lanka and is dated from between 1771 and 1910.

This will include further questioning, followed by a physical examination of the eyes, nose, tongue, nails, feet, skin and hair.

What type of treatment is given?

Treatment is given not just for the condition but also to improve your whole life. Diet and lifestyle changes will be advised, as well as medication. First, there must be a detoxification of the body. This could involve massage with oils (*Purvakarma*), followed by sweat therapy (*Swedanakarma*) to eliminate wastes from the body. Internal detoxification (*Panchakarma*) to remove toxins from the body involves emetics, fasting and steam inhalations.

Sometimes rejuvenation therapy (*Rasayana*) may be necessary for a long-term illness. This aims to boost the immune system and mental faculties. Yoga, meditation and counselling may also be advised. Natural herbal remedies will then be prescribed. These have been in use for thousands of years and evaluated within the Ayurvedic philosophy, but many of them are also known and used in the West. The Indian and Sri Lankan governments fund on-going research into Ayurvedic medicine and, because of the interest in the West, many drug companies are also conducting research. The Ayurvedic medical authorities keep updated databases on the results of such research and this can be referred to by fully qualified practitioners.

Can Ayurvedic medicine improve energy levels?

In Ayurvedic medicine, *marma* therapy is used to influence body functions. It works like acupressure, relating specific disorders to points on the body. Lack of energy relates to a point situated at the top of the head, which is also associated with headaches, migraine and memory problems. Applying gentle pressure to the point energises it or depresses it, depending on which is required. However, a practitioner will also

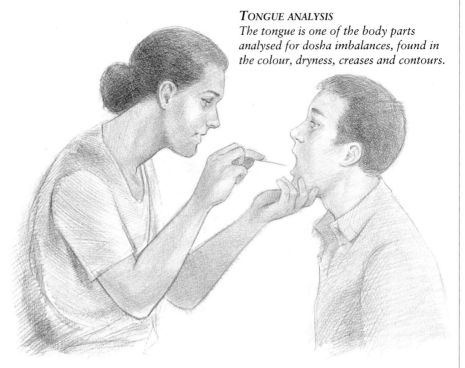

TONGUE ANALYSIS
The tongue is one of the body parts analysed for dosha imbalances, found in the colour, dryness, creases and contours.

advise on an energising diet specific to your dosha type and your lifestyle to further promote energy.

What can Ayurvedic medicine treat?

Ayurvedic medicine works as a complement to orthodox medicine. Practitioners aim to support Western medicine, rather than replace it, and so it can treat a range of disorders.

However, it has been found to be particularly suitable for conditions such as irritable bowel syndrome, ME, flu, depression, insomnia, anxiety, asthma, joint conditions such as arthritis and osteoarthritis, and a wide range of skin conditions such as eczema and dermatitis.

How are the practitioners qualified?

In India practitioners learn from a fully qualified teacher or attend a five-year course. There are few opportunities for training in the UK.

WHAT YOU CAN DO AT HOME

Most Ayurvedic medicine must be prescribed by a practitioner, although there are simple remedies that can treat minor illnesses.

Headaches and sinus problems

Boil 4 tablespoons of coriander seeds in water for 10 minutes, place in a bowl and then inhale the steam to clear the nasal passages.

Colds

Gently brown 4 tablespoons of coriander seeds in a pan, add 4 cups of water and 4 slices of ginger root and boil. Reduce by half its volume, strain and drink.

Indigestion

Slice some fresh root ginger and then chew thoroughly to extract the juice. Swallow the juice and discard the chewed pulp.

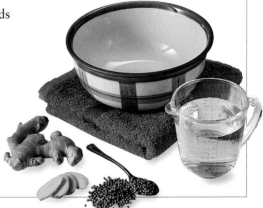

the occurrences during that year and the nature of the people born in that year. Your animal and your element are used to find your strengths and weaknesses and predict your destiny. They are frequently used to explain relationships and compatibility between friends and family. The diagram on page 49 shows how each element relates to the others: each controls one element and feeds another, all interlinking and working as a whole system.

The Chinese take their astrology very seriously and many follow the predictions with great fervour. The compatibility of marriage partnerships is often determined according to astrological links. Couples frequently plan their children to fall within certain years – the most popular being the year of the Dragon, with the year of the Snake coming a close second. Some years are also avoided: traditionally, female babies born in the year of the Fire Horse (which occurs once in every 60 years) were killed at birth because it was felt that they were too rebellious and uncontrollable to suit the traditional female temperament.

THE FIVE ELEMENTS AND CHINESE ASTROLOGY

Your astrological animal and element are indicated by the year in which you were born. If, however, you were born in January (before the Chinese new year) you will be part of the previous year. The characteristics of the astrological animals are given in the table below. For a description of your element, see the diagram on page 49. The animal describes your character tendencies, whereas the element explains your deeper emotional status and the relationships with those around you. The animal and element of the current year are used for predictions of future events, and how you may be put out of balance by the changing energy forces. Advice often focuses on diet and behavioural changes to rebalance your energies and avoid misfortune.

ELEMENT	METAL	FIRE	WATER	EARTH	WOOD	CHARACTERISTICS
Rat	1900 1960	1936 1996	1912 1972	1948 2008	1924 1984	Restless, aggressive, charming, successful, discontented, expressive, perfectionist, stubborn, adamant
Ox	1901 1961	1937 1997	1913 1973	1949 2009	1925 1985	Diligent, patient, observant, good memory, dogmatic, hard-working, practical, strong-willed
Tiger	1902 1962	1938 1998	1914 1974	1950 2010	1926 1986	Powerful, leader, daring, magnetic, confident, authoritative, good fighter, warm-hearted, dominating, egotistical
Rabbit	1903 1963	1939 1999	1915 1975	1951 2011	1927 1987	Delicate, kind, loving, popular, cool, conservative, insecure, pessimistic, well-dressed, lovable, peaceful, sensitive, lucky
Dragon	1904 1964	1940 2000	1916 1976	1952 2012	1928 1988	Noble, masterful, powerful, perfectionist, influential, dynamic, inflexible, lucky, idealist, stubborn, forceful
Snake	1905 1965	1941 2001	1917 1977	1953 2013	1929 1989	Diplomatic, charming, popular, deep-thinking, intellectual, intuitive, perceptive, thoughtful, inspired, charismatic, ostentatious
Horse	1906 1966	1942 2002	1918 1978	1954 2014	1930 1990	Energetic, hot-blooded, rebellious, impatient, quick-witted, cunning, selfish, productive, sociable, capable, independent
Goat	1907 1967	1943 2003	1919 1979	1955 2015	1931 1991	Gentle, elegant, creative, charming, dreamers, lazy, insecure, pessimistic, relaxed, self-centred, lovable
Monkey	1908 1968	1944 2004	1920 1980	1956 2016	1932 1992	Merry, fun, loving, cheerful, generous, deceptive, clever, diplomatic, creative, sociable, carefree, energetic
Rooster	1909 1969	1945 2005	1921 1981	1957 2017	1933 1993	Enthusiastic, observant, accurate, attention-seeking, cautious, perceptive, analysing, resourceful, practical
Dog	1910 1970	1946 2006	1922 1982	1958 2018	1934 1994	Dutiful, honest, faithful, sincere, honourable, loyal, caring, defensive, judgmental, loving, jealous, amicable
Pig	1911 1971	1947 2007	1923 1983	1959 2019	1935 1995	Chivalrous, sincere, tolerant, honourable, admirable, loving, generous, companionable, obliging, thoughtful, considerate

CHAPTER 3

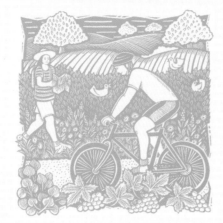

ENERGY DRAINERS

Everyday lifestyle factors can have a significant influence on your energy levels. Increasing your awareness of how you are affected by your working and living environments, your emotional state, your dietary habits, even your use of common drugs such as caffeine or aspirin, can help you to maximise your energy and improve your health.

SLEEP AND ENERGY

The duration and quality of your sleep has a profound effect on your daytime performance, as well as on your health, happiness and, indeed, the whole quality of your life.

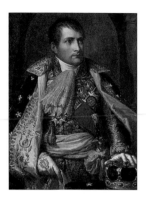

*SLEEPING PATTERNS
Napoleon regularly slept for less than five hours each night. However, he slept for 36 hours after his defeat in the Battle of Aspern in 1809, the first battle that the French Emperor lost after 17 successive triumphs.*

Sleep plays an essential part in the body's daily routine. It allows the body to rest tired muscles, restore depleted energy levels and carry out repairs to the tissues. Sleep also allows the conscious mind to rest and recuperate, and enables the unconscious mind to store the skills and knowledge acquired during the day. The young of all species sleep longer than the adults and the amount of sleep that individuals need diminishes with age, suggesting that sleep may be particularly important for growth, development and learning.

REVITALISING YOUR BODY
As you drift off to sleep, your muscles become more relaxed, your heartbeat and breathing rate slow down, your blood pressure drops and your temperature falls. The digestive system remains active, although your metabolic rate decreases by around 20 per cent. Some senses, such as hearing, continue to monitor any changes in your surroundings, but the deeper the sleep the less responsive the brain becomes to these external stimuli. All these processes are important for the proper rest and recuperation of body and mind, encouraging energy renewal and alertness during waking hours.

On average, adults need about eight hours' sleep, although this figure drops to around four to six hours in old age. Sleep requirements vary from person to person and from day to day, however, depending on the individual's sex, activity levels and environment, as well as genetic and general health factors. Many people need more or less than the average amount as a matter of course, or on particular days of the week.

Too little sleep is a common problem, affecting daytime energy levels, as well as physical health and psychological well-being. Generally, a longer sleep provides a deeper sleep, allowing the body to recuperate more completely. Poor, unrefreshing sleep is considered by some doctors as a significant factor in myalgic encephalomyelitis, or ME, an increasingly common condition also known as chronic fatigue syndrome.

Energy levels can also be affected by too much sleep. It has been found that excessive sleep can lead to fatigue, lack of motivation, a loss of alertness and an inability to make decisions. Many people with ME find that regularly sleeping for more than 11 hours a day can worsen their symptoms. In these cases, restricting sleep to an average of eight to nine hours may help to reduce fatigue.

Having an irregular sleep pattern can also lead to daytime symptoms such as fatigue and difficulty concentrating. Changes in sleep pattern between weekdays and weekends is thought by sleep disorder specialists to contribute to the general feeling of lethargy known as the 'Monday morning feeling'. Sleep and disease are intricately related and

SLEEP AND AGE

Babies start to have a regular sleeping pattern from about six months onwards, although they rarely sleep for long periods. As people get older, they need less sleep, but they also have more problems associated with sleeplessness.

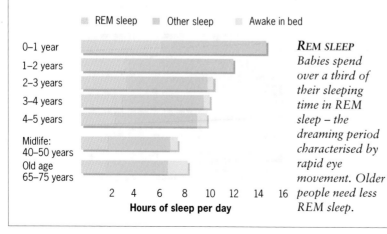

■ REM sleep   ■ Other sleep   ■ Awake in bed

0–1 year
1–2 years
2–3 years
3–4 years
4–5 years
Midlife:
40–50 years
Old age
65–75 years

2   4   6   8   10   12   14   16
Hours of sleep per day

*REM SLEEP
Babies spend over a third of their sleeping time in REM sleep – the dreaming period characterised by rapid eye movement. Older people need less REM sleep.*

excessive drowsiness may be a symptom of serious illness, for example a brain disorder or head injury such as subdural bleeding, hormonal problems, or liver failure.

SLEEP DISORDERS

Sleep apnoea, or heavy snoring, is a relatively common disorder that often goes undetected. The most common type, obstructive sleep apnoea, mainly affects overweight men between the ages of 30 and 50. The heavy snoring is usually caused by an obstruction to the passage of air from enlarged tonsils or adenoids, or over-relaxation of the muscles in the soft palate.

Other types of sleep apnoea are caused by disorders of the brain or diaphragm, or a mixture of causes. The condition can usually be alleviated by sleeping on your side or front to keep the airway open (see pages 58–59). Alcohol and sleeping drugs should be avoided as they can aggravate sleep apnoea. Pickwickian Syndrome, a condition named after a character in Charles Dickens'

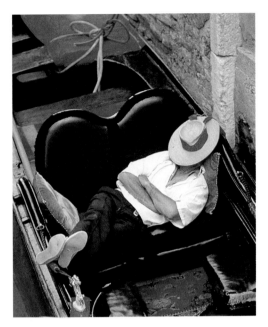

Pickwick Papers, involves a combination of sleep apnoea, extreme obesity and constant sleepiness. The cause is unknown, although it is improved by weight loss.

INSOMNIA

Insomnia is the term used to describe sleep problems such as difficulty falling asleep, repeated waking, and early waking before the sleep cycle is complete. It is a common complaint, experienced by around 40 per cent of adults at some time in their lives. Insufficient or disturbed sleep commonly leads to aching and tired muscles and feelings of lethargy the following day. It can be caused by a number of factors, including pain, noise or discomfort, stress, or hormonal changes, such as those that occur during pregnancy. Most cases of insomnia are temporary and do not pose a significant threat to health. However, long-term insomnia can seriously affect the sufferer's quality of life and professional medical help should be sought. In some cases sleeping pills may provide temporary relief, but medication seldom provides a long-term solution as it can interfere with sleep patterns and lead to drug tolerance, requiring progressively larger doses to achieve the same effect.

HYPERSOMNIA AND NARCOLEPSY

Hypersomnia, or excessive sleep, can cause daytime drowsiness. This is a recognised medical problem: hypersomniacs are lacking in energy and enthusiasm and run the risk of becoming caffeine or amphetamine addicts to keep themselves awake.

In most women there is evidence of minor sleep changes with the menstrual cycle and during pregnancy. These changes are not specifically attributed to changes in sex hormone levels, although periodic hypersomnia has been linked to menstruation since 1943 when the first case was reported in a 14-year-old girl. She slept deeply for four or five days, beginning on the fourth day of her menstrual cycle; when awake, the girl ate excessively. A number of similar examples of menstrual hypersomnolence have since been reported though not always featuring overeating. Hypersomnia during menstruation may cease when ovulation is stopped by oral contraceptive pills.

Chronic intake of drugs and alcohol can also cause hypersomnia and lethargy. This is because stimulants alter the brain's normal sleep patterns leading to disturbed sleep and sleep apnoea. In people who already suffer sleep disorders, excessive intake of alcohol and drugs can exacerbate the disorders and lead to further problems.

TIPS ON AVOIDING INSOMNIA

Here are some techniques that may help to combat insomnia:

▶ *Develop a regular bedtime routine.*

▶ *No matter how tired you feel, don't lie in bed later than normal.*

▶ *Avoid heavy meals and excess alcohol too late in the evening.*

▶ *Have a warm, caffeine-free drink and a biscuit before bed.*

▶ *Sprinkle a few drops of lavender oil on your pillow.*

▶ *Have a warm bath with relaxing aromatherapy oils.*

▶ *Take exercise at least three times a week.*

▶ *Learn a relaxation technique such as deep breathing which you can do at bedtime.*

▶ *Don't lie in bed worrying – if you can't sleep, get up and do something else until you feel more sleepy.*

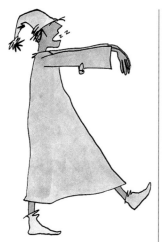

MOBILE SLEEPER
Sleepwalking can be a frightening experience. Although it is not dangerous to wake a sleepwalker, it is sensible to guide him or her gently back to bed while still sleeping.

An extreme, but rare, form of persistent daytime drowsiness is called narcolepsy, which causes the sufferer to fall asleep repeatedly throughout the day. Sufferers may also experience sudden muscle collapse, called cataplexy, as well as hallucinations and dreams while awake. The disorder is often inherited and can be highly disruptive to a person's life. It is usually treated with medication and regular naps.

OTHER SLEEP DISORDERS

Sleepwalking, or somnambulism, occurs when a sleeping person gets out of bed and moves around without waking. Up to 25 per cent of people experience this at least once in their lives, usually in childhood. It most often affects children between five and ten years old and is usually outgrown by the age of 15. A related disorder, night terrors, occurs when a person, normally a young child, awakens from a deep sleep with a sense of great fear, pounding pulse and laboured breathing. Most people grow out of these traumatic experiences and those who reach adulthood and are still having night terrors often seek help to find the underlying cause of the problem.

JET LAG

Long-distance air travel that crosses several time zones causes people to change their normal sleep patterns. Travellers suddenly have to fit in with meal and sleep times of a different country, while their internal body clock is still working to the time pattern of the country they have just left. In most people the result is jet lag, a condition that causes similar symptoms to shiftwork: sleepiness and fatigue during the waking period and insomnia during the sleep period. The severity of the condition increases according to the number of time zones crossed. Regular travellers usually find that westbound flights are less disruptive than eastbound flights due to the westward movement of the sun.

Both sleepwalking and night terrors differ from dreams or nightmares in that they occur during deep sleep periods, and not during the REM phase. The cause is unknown although they are more common

SLEEP PATTERNS

As you fall asleep, you pass through various stages of sleep which are categorised according to the level of brain activity. The lightest sleep occurs just after you have fallen asleep and dreaming is done during this period, known as the rapid eye movement (REM) stage because of the visible eye movements that take place as you dream. The next four stages take you to progressively deeper sleep until you reach the deepest level, stage 4. During a normal sleep period you pass from stage 1 to stage 4 and back again several times without waking up. As you go through the lighter sleep stages you pass through REM sleep, possibly a few times a night in an average sleep. The longer that you spend asleep, the shorter are the periods of deep sleep and the longer the lighter, REM dream periods, which is why people often wake up dreaming.

SLEEP CHART
When you go to sleep at night, your body gradually goes into deep sleep, through REM sleep (coloured yellow) and the four stages. You may remain in deep sleep for a period before returning to light sleep. The graph below shows the progression of a normal night's sleep for an average sleeper over a seven-hour period.

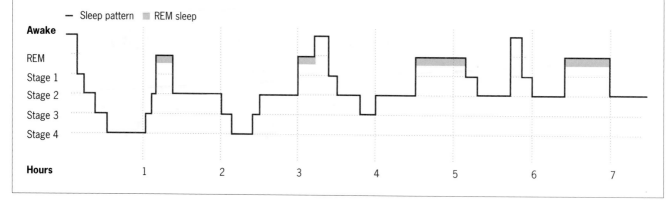

during times of anxiety and stress and tend to run in families. If the condition is persistent you should seek professional help.

ALTERED SLEEP PATTERNS

In some situations, usually work-related, people have to adopt unnatural sleep patterns. A common example of this is shiftwork, which has long been an accepted pattern of working life for many people. It has been estimated that up to a third of male workers and a fifth of female workers do some form of shiftwork rotation.

In occupations such as security and some factory jobs, staff may work continual night shifts. This requires a major adjustment to the normal sleep cycle as it involves sleeping during the day, when the body is naturally at its most active, and working at night when the body would normally be at rest.

THE EFFECTS OF DREAMING

On average, dreaming occurs four or five times during the night, in sessions lasting 5–20 minutes. It is thought that deprivation of dream sleep can lead to learning problems in children and psychological difficulties in adults. People who do not get enough dream sleep often suffer reduced alertness and vitality. In experiments, people who

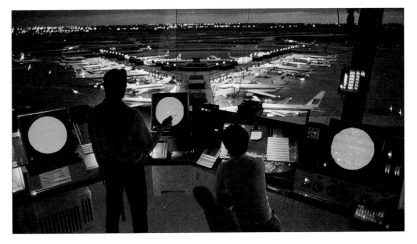

have been deprived of dream sleep become irritable, lose concentration and may even hallucinate. Subsequent sleep periods contain a higher than normal proportion of dream sleep to enable thcm to catch up. A lack of dream sleep can also occur as a result of taking sleeping pills or drugs; they can keep the mind in a state of deep sleep and prevent proper REM dream stages which are necessary for the mind to sort out problems and deal with emotions.

Dream periods become longer and more frequent according to the length of time that is spent asleep. Babies and young children, who spend much more time asleep than adults, have longer periods of dream sleep, and this has been linked to mental development and the promotion of brain activity. Although the actual purpose of dreams has never been proved, many psychologists believe that the subconscious – the instinctive part of the mind that is hidden from the conscious, rational mind – expresses itself through dreams, helping individuals to work through complex emotional and psychological problems. A range of therapies, especially the psychiatric therapies, use dream analysis to uncover a person's problems and frustrations.

Some people remember their dreams very vividly, while others rarely realise that they have dreamt at all during the night. Most people, however, experience nightmares at some point during their lives, when they are awoken by an unpleasant dream with a powerful emotional content of anxiety, terror, or dread of death. Nightmares occur most often in childhood when the REM periods are longer and more frequent. As people age they become more adapted to their experiences and need to dream less.

ALCOHOL AND SLEEP

Alcohol can severely disrupt the quality of sleep. Research has shown that going to bed after drinking sends you quickly into a deep sleep, but when the sedating effect of the alcohol wears off, you may wake up and find it difficult to get to sleep again. Small doses of drinking are fine and can help you to relax, but any more than a couple of glasses of wine or beer can lead to sleeping problems. A typical result is deep sleep for three to four hours, followed by recurrent waking with sweating, headaches, intense dreams or nightmares. Long-term sleeping problems due to alcoholism will have a marked effect on energy levels and mental well-being. In heavy drinkers, abstinence can also cause insomnia. For sound sleep, it is best to drink alcohol moderately or not at all.

SHIFTWORK
Up to 80 per cent of shiftworkers suffer serious sleep-related disorders, typically drowsiness and lethargy at work and insomnia at home. There is little doubt that people function best in the usual 24-hour cycle, and that in all shiftwork situations, performance, concentration and decision-making tend to suffer.

Dealing with

Snoring

Snoring affects not just individual sufferers – those around them, especially their partners, may also be prevented from getting a good night's sleep. The inevitable result is daytime tiredness, a loss of concentration and vitality, and irritability.

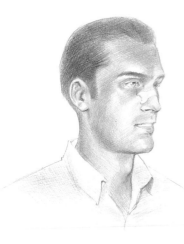

DEVICES THAT STOP SNORING
This lightweight nose plaster pulls open the nasal passages, allowing you to breathe more easily through your upper nose. They are available from chemists and are relatively inexpensive.

Snoring occurs when the tissues inside the nose and throat partially block the windpipe, preventing easy breathing. Sleep apnoea is a more serious snoring condition that occurs when the tissues lose their tone and become flabby, leading to a blockage of the airways. The result of both of these conditions is that breathing becomes blocked or disjointed, and is often prevented completely for a number of seconds before the brain triggers a gasping or snorting response to restore breathing. This response usually wakes the sleeper slightly, which opens the airways once again and the whole process restarts. Getting a good night's sleep becomes difficult after these persistent disruptions, and sufferers inevitably find themselves feeling tired and lacking in energy.

Snoring is more likely to affect people over the age of 30 as muscle tone reduces with age. Other conditions can also contribute to snoring, such as a tumour or cyst in the airway.

LIVING WITH A SNORING PROBLEM

There are a number of precautions you can take to help to reduce or relieve snoring. Adapting your lifestyle and becoming more health-conscious will help most cases of apnoea and snoring, although more serious cases often need larger lifestyle adjustments. Corrective surgery can be done to remove or 'tuck' the tissue that is causing the problem, although doctors usually only resort to this if the condition is so severe that it has become dangerous.

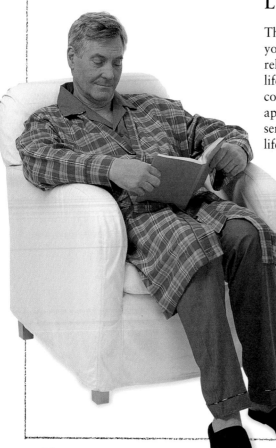

DON'T STRAIN YOURSELF
Going to bed over-tired or absolutely exhausted can compound a snoring problem by relaxing your muscles and tissues and allowing them to block your airways. Avoid fatigue by taking rests during the day and make sure that you go to bed on time every night.

▶ *If you are overweight, slimming down usually helps apnoea dramatically. A study in the United States has found that a 10 to 25 per cent drop in weight significantly improves snoring problems and apnoea. This is because the excess weight puts pressure on the tissues and encourages sagging.*

▶ *Give up cigarette smoking as this can often cause inflammation of the airways and also increase the mucus production in the nasal passages.*

▶ *Moderate your intake of alcohol as it over-relaxes the muscles and tissues.*

▶ *Make sure that you get a good night's sleep every night. Going to bed over-tired will over-relax the muscles, making them sag and therefore interfere with your proper breathing.*

▶ *Reduce the stress in your life by taking up a relaxation routine.*

▶ *Relax before going to bed, by sitting quietly or having a warm bath. If you are not relaxed when you go to bed, there is more chance that your tissues will over-relax and exacerbate your snoring.*

HELPING TO PREVENT SNORING

Staying asleep at night can be difficult if you suffer from apnoea. Some sufferers, on the other hand, find that they sleep throughout the night but still wake up tired because snoring has prevented them from entering a deep sleep. Try one or several of the techniques below to prevent snoring.

▶ *Keep your evening meals light and don't eat too much just before you go to bed. Heavy food can over-relax you, causing your tissues and muscles to lose tone and interfere with your airways.*

▶ *Raise your head and shoulders above the bed with a firm pillow, preferably holding your jaw away from your body. Try sleeping on an incline by tilting the whole bed with boards or bricks under the legs at the head of the bed. This will open the airways and allow you to breathe normally.*

▶ *Clear your nose and throat properly before you go to bed. Special nasal sprays can be bought from most chemists.*

▶ *Sleep on your stomach or your side. Sleeping on your back tends to aggravate snoring problems as most of the blockages are caused by the front of the throat and nasal passages relaxing downwards.*

▶ *Special sleeping masks fitted over the mouth and nose by a doctor can keep air pressure at a level that prevents the airways from blocking. They are known as 'continuous positive airway pressure machines' and are very effective, although impractical for many users.*

▶ *A variety of dental devices can be used to keep your tongue away from your throat and your jaw forwards to prevent airway blockage. A doctor or orthodontist needs to advise you and fit such devices.*

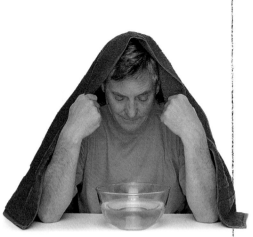

CLEARING YOUR PASSAGES
Make sure your nose and throat are clear of phlegm and mucus so they do not disrupt your breathing through the night. Nasal sprays and inhalations can both be used, as well as herbal inhalations.

SLEEPING WITH SOMEONE WITH A SNORING PROBLEM

If your partner has a severe snoring problem, you may find that your own sleep is suffering, perhaps more than your partner's, leaving you tired and agitated in the morning and putting a strain on your relationship. There are a number of steps you can take to ease the problem, although preventing the snoring altogether with one or other of the suggestions above would be the best solution as it would also help your partner sleep better through the night.

▶ *Try gently pinching your partner's nose closed with your finger and thumb. It may encourage your partner to move into a better breathing position.*

▶ *If you can't stop the noise, try wearing ear-plugs so that you can't hear it.*

▶ *Concentrating on something else, or sometimes even concentrating on the snoring, can help you to forget that it is preventing you from sleeping.*

▶ *Go to sleep before your partner does so that you are already asleep when he or she starts to snore.*

CAUTION
Be careful when taking medications for snoring because they often prevent you from entering deep sleep, leaving you tired the following day. Likewise, if your partner's snoring is keeping you awake at night, sleeping pills are not a viable long-term solution.

Raise the snorer's head to stop blockages in the throat

Move the snorer onto his or her side or front to help to prevent snoring

THE CORRECT POSITION
Make sure that your partner sleeps in the right position, on his or her side with the head slightly raised to open the air passages.

EMOTIONAL DRAIN ON ENERGY

Emotional problems are among the most widespread underlying causes of fatigue. Disorders stemming from overwork, grief, pressure or anxiety can quickly deplete your energy levels.

Low energy levels resulting from emotional problems, at any stage of life, no matter what the cause, tend to share certain key features; activity levels slow down and there is a reluctance to start even the most basic tasks. Physical activities, especially exercise, are avoided. Social intercourse becomes unattractive and the individual quickly loses interest in even the pleasurable activities, including sex. This can have a knock-on effect on the hormone system, leaving sufferers less able to motivate themselves.

DEPRESSION

Depressive illness has been recognised for over 2000 years and, according to some experts, is the cause of more human misery than any other single disease. Depression accounts for an estimated 50 per cent of psychiatric disorders and more than 10 per cent of all visits to GP surgeries. Clinical depression is a severe manifestation of the problem and may require hospitalisation in some cases. Depression is often associated with a multitude of symptoms, including low spirits, irritability, lack of motivation,

HOW DRUGS CAN AFFECT YOUR EMOTIONS

Neurons in the brain communicate to each other by means of neurotransmitters. These tiny chemicals are released from one neuron, pass through the synaptic gap where their presence is experienced as a feeling, and are received into another neuron. Drugs have been developed to alter mood through the control of neurotransmitter efficiency. This is done through three main techniques: by increasing the synthesis or production of neurotransmitters, by increasing the release of neurotransmitters, or by releasing replica neurotransmitters which have a similar effect on the nervous system.

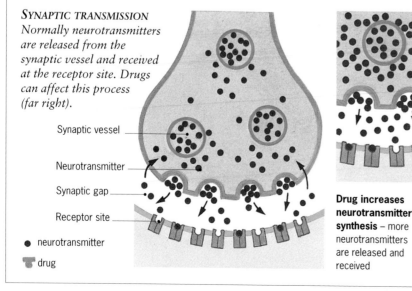

SYNAPTIC TRANSMISSION
Normally neurotransmitters are released from the synaptic vessel and received at the receptor site. Drugs can affect this process (far right).

Synaptic vessel

Neurotransmitter

Synaptic gap

Receptor site

• neurotransmitter

⊤ drug

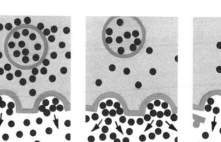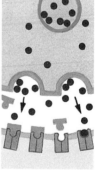

Drug increases neurotransmitter synthesis – more neurotransmitters are released and received

Drug increases release of neurotransmitters into the synaptic gap and more are therefore received

Drug contains artificial neurotransmitters which activate receptor sites just like natural ones do

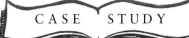

The Perfectionist

Placing too many or too exacting demands on yourself can exhaust you both mentally and physically, reducing your energy levels and preventing you from functioning healthily. Clearing your head and taking time to relax can help you to get your life back into perspective, giving you the energy you need for a full and happy life.

Sebastian, 26, has always been a perfectionist. He is also ambitious and has been working very hard at a postgraduate doctorate in economics. Recently, however, he has felt insecure about his work, especially after a progress meeting with his tutor who suggested that parts of his thesis lacked depth. He has been working all hours researching and rewriting his thesis, and drinking too much coffee to help him to stay alert. He is constantly tired but has difficulty sleeping. His girlfriend, Gail, has become increasingly concerned that he asks too much of himself. She thinks he has done enough to earn the doctorate, but Sebastian feels his work can still be improved and cannot let it go.

WHAT SHOULD SEBASTIAN DO?

Gail suggested that Sebastian try rational emotive therapy to help him put his perfectionist urges into perspective. This therapy looks for the underlying causes of obsessive attitudes and actions so that they can be addressed and resolved. The therapist will ask Sebastian about his views on work, status and achievement, as well as his upbringing, his own sense of self-worth and performance anxieties. Together they can work through Sebastian's inner anxieties and his expectations of both himself and those around him. The therapist can then make suggestions as to how he can tackle these anxieties, especially his negative reaction to criticism and his inability to relax.

STRESS
Striving too hard for perfection, or taking too much on, can cause you to lose sight of your own personal goals.

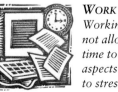

WORK
Working too hard and not allowing enough time to enjoy other aspects of life can lead to stress build-up.

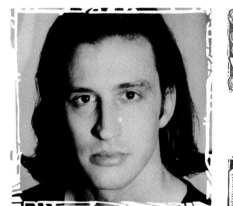

EMOTIONS
Many energy problems are caused by emotional problems that need to be resolved.

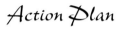

Action Plan

STRESS
Take time off to relax, using meditation and yoga techniques. Spend time doing fun activities to get more from life.

WORK
Don't overwork – take a break rather than working non-stop for hours at a time. Learn to be more realistic about goals and deadlines.

EMOTIONS
Consider the reasons underlying behaviour. Are they appropriate? Do they reflect own dreams or someone else's?

HOW THINGS TURNED OUT FOR SEBASTIAN

The rational emotive therapist quickly realised that Sebastian's perfectionism stemmed from his upbringing. The therapist helped him to see that he was unconsciously holding on to old behavioural patterns of demanding parental approval, which he no longer needed as an adult. He was encouraged to take up yoga, both to help him to relax and to increase his energy. He successfully completed his doctorate.

Finding your own path

Many parents have great ambitions for their children, although these often reflect goals that they themselves could not achieve, or the desire to maintain a family business, profession or status. Identifying and pursuing your own ambitions is one of life's greatest challenges.

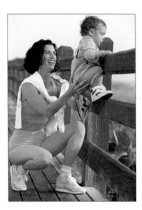

A GUIDING HAND
The guidance that parents give their children should be helpful in encouraging them to stand on their own feet.

poor concentration and sleep problems, but it invariably includes fatigue and a general lack of energy.

Depression can often occur as a reaction to a stressful situation that a person cannot cope with. This is called reactive depression. Grieving in response to the death of a spouse, for example, can include strong depressive feelings. Another example is the depression that follows a stroke or other serious physical illness. Depression is also common after childbirth, the so-called 'baby blues', or can be a characteristic of hormonal disturbances, such as in premenstrual syndrome. When depression occurs for no known reason it is called endogenous. This form of depression tends to run in families and affects around 20 per cent of women and 10 per cent of men.

STRESS AND ANXIETY

A limited degree of stress and tension in life is beneficial and can actually boost energy levels and performance, helping to motivate individuals and spur them on to greater levels of achievement. But excessive stress and anxiety sap energy, eating away at the person's vitality. They can create an energy vacuum, leading to poor health, greater anxiety and a downward spiral of fatigue and low self-esteem that prevents the sufferer from leading a normal and happy life.

One reason for this may be that prolonged stress can induce biological changes in a part of the brain called the hypothalamus

ENERGY BOOST

Spring cleaning – even in the winter months – can be fun and energising, brushing away the old cobwebs and making space for new pursuits and ideas. An interesting complementary therapy is space-clearing, involving the spiritual cleansing of a room by clapping the hands together and ringing out the bad energy, neutralising it for your own thoughts, ambitions and enjoyment. Space-clearing enables you to fill your personal space with positive feelings, building the foundations for an energised life.

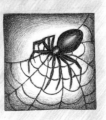

which, together with the pituitary gland, regulates hormone levels and autonomic functions such as heart and breathing rate. The feelings of being hungry and of being satiated, and the sensations of warmth and cold are located at specific centres in the hypothalamus, and it is now believed that similar centres exist there for rest and fatigue. When the hypothalamus-pituitary system is disturbed by stress or depression, there is a consequent disruption in the normal regime of activity and rest, resulting in fatigue, lethargy and an inability to sleep.

OVERWORK AND 'BURNOUT'

In today's society, the pressure to succeed is becoming a major cause of stress and stress-related disorders, and can ultimately lead to chronic fatigue and an inability to function. Greater competition and increased media coverage of success, high achievers and status symbols serve as inducements to push people to their limits. Stress can manifest itself as a physical stress-related condition, such as digestive problems, or nerve disorders such as mental breakdown.

Mental relaxation training is an important step to overcome or avoid the build-up of chronic stress. Relaxation techniques encourage a positive response to excess stress by decreasing heart rate and slowing down breathing. Yoga is a form of exercise practised for mental relaxation and it may help to relieve disorders such as insomnia which can often be stress related.

Taking exercise and concentrating on your physical abilities can be surprisingly good for stress relief. Take your frustration out in a challenging squash competition or strenuous aerobics class. Making fitness fun and inspiring can lift your spirits and help you to overcome stress and emotional problems. Try a new dance class, or play a game of rounders in the park with friends.

Burnout

Burnout is a state of exhaustion in which you feel unable to do anything and have a variety of aches and illnesses. It is most often a result of trying too hard at one thing to the exclusion of all else, and can be countered with relaxation and time off.

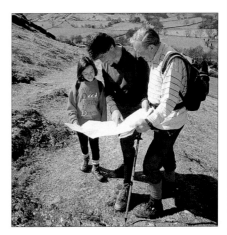

GET AWAY FROM IT ALL
Taking time off and getting away from your day-to-day life can help you to get problems and pressures back into perspective.

Many people suffer from burnout at some point in their lives to a lesser or greater degree, although sometimes they may not realise it themselves. Burnout occurs when your body is telling you that you need change. You have been working too hard at one part of your life, often your job, and neglecting everything else. A human being needs a balance between the emotional, social, intellectual and practical sides: the denial or neglect of one leads to an imbalance which resounds throughout the whole. Many people suffering from burnout are perfectionists at their work and feel that they are not getting enough support and appreciation from others, often because of isolation. The warning signs include unexplained tiredness, irritability, difficulties in socialising and relaxing, and feelings of disenchantment, disorientation, cynicism or sadness.

HELPING TO COPE WITH BURNOUT

There are a number of things you can do to reduce the risk of burnout, or methods to help you cope if it does strike you down.

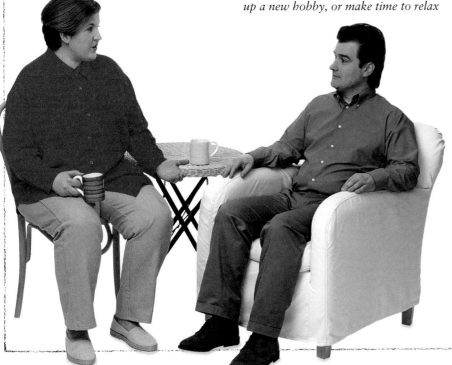

▶ *First of all you need to admit that you have a problem. Make a conscious effort to change and focus on a number of measures to help you.*

▶ *Bring more variety into your life. Take up a new hobby, or make time to relax with friends. Get away for a few days, even if it's not far from your home. Take some fresh air and get some exercise. It is important to have a part of your life that is not goal orientated.*

▶ *Stop being a perfectionist by understanding that people do make mistakes and need time and energy for a variety of things in life. Don't be a slave to your work or your goals.*

▶ *Accept your personal and emotional needs and limitations. If you need support or feedback, admit it to yourself and find the support that you need.*

▶ *Practise relaxation exercises (see Chapter 5) and take a break frequently to remind yourself what life is about in a wider context.*

TALK TO YOUR FAMILY AND FRIENDS
Many problems concerned with burnout can be positively addressed by opening up to someone close, who can also be given the opportunity to share his or her worries. Self-expression is one of the keys to good emotional health.

ALLERGIES AND INTOLERANCES

Occurring at any time of life, allergies and intolerances often cause fatigue and a loss of vitality. The situation may be compounded by difficulties in correctly diagnosing the cause.

THE MAIN SUSPECTS

The most usual triggers for allergic reactions are:

▶ *Plant pollens or mould spores in the air.*

▶ *Milk, dairy products or nuts in the diet.*

▶ *Animal hair or dirt in the air or on skin contact.*

▶ *Drugs such as antibiotics and penicillin.*

▶ *Dust mites and insect bites or stings.*

▶ *Cosmetics on the skin.*

Allergies and intolerances are common medical problems which can cause a wide range of symptoms, including fatigue. An allergy is an abnormal reaction by the immune system to substances that are perfectly harmless to other people. The immune system's function is to recognise antigens (foreign proteins) and form antibodies to destroy them. Allergic reactions occur when the immune system mistakes a harmless substance for an antigen and builds up an army of antibodies to destroy it. This hypersensitivity can be a highly exaggerated response and can sometimes be very dangerous. An intolerance is also an abnormal reaction to a harmless substance, but it does not involve the immune system.

Some reactions are easy to diagnose because they occur in very specific situations or at particular times of year. One example is hayfever which a sufferer may notice is triggered by grass pollen and only occurs in the

DID YOU KNOW?

Around half of all food intolerance sufferers have a strange addiction to the food that makes them unwell. This is thought to be because the allergen has a side effect that increases the activity of endorphins – the brain's natural painkillers – stimulating a good feeling. Intolerances to dairy or wheat products often cause this addiction.

AVOIDING HIGH POLLEN COUNTS

Many people are allergic to pollen and understanding how and when different types of pollen are dispersed can help sufferers to control an allergy. Tree pollen counts soar in May, grasses through June and July, and weed pollen is rife during August and September. Pollen levels also vary greatly throughout the day.

POLLEN LEVELS THROUGH THE DAY
Pollen is released in the morning and carried high in the air until late afternoon, when it falls back to the ground, sometimes many miles away. Hayfever sufferers are warned against outdoor pursuits in the afternoon when the pollen is returning to the ground.

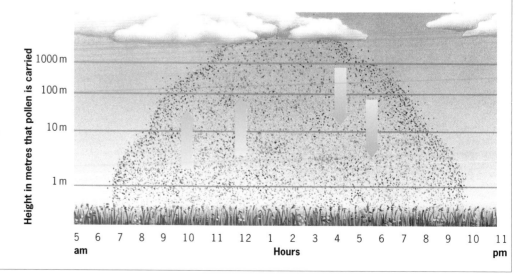

ALLERGIC TENSION-FATIGUE SYNDROME

This theory, developed in the US in the 1930s, proposes that repeated exposure to an allergen exhausts the body, including the immune system, and leaves it open to illness and further medical complications. This can have a degenerative effect on energy levels, leading to chronic fatigue and serious health problems. Removing the allergen will improve not only the symptoms of the allergy but also the medical conditions caused by the drain on energy levels.

ALLERGIC DISORDERS AND FATIGUE

Many symptoms can be the result of an undetected allergy, although there are often a number of potential causes for each illness, condition or symptom. Allergies are one of the commonest causes of fatigue problems, but they can often remain hidden for years. The culprits may be identified by using an allergy diary and testing for reactions.

SYMPTOM	POSSIBLE CAUSE
Skin inflammation, eczema or dermatitis	House dust mites, washing powders, soaps, creams, cosmetics, fabrics, stress, foods
Respiratory problems, wheezing, asthma	Pollen, house dust mites, airborne dirt or dust particles, pet hairs, mould spores, chemical fumes, food
Gastrointestinal disorders, vomiting, diarrhoea, colic	Food or drinks, materials from cooking utensils, stress
Genitourinary disorders, candida, cystitis	Tight or unaerated clothing, washing powders, soaps, food and drink

summer. In many cases, particularly where food is concerned, the cause of an allergy or intolerance can be difficult to establish.

SYMPTOMS OF FOOD ALLERGY

Allergies and intolerances can cause a mixed and often confusing range of symptoms, including nausea, vomiting, headaches, skin rash, migraine, ulcers, sinusitis, asthma, and muscle, bone and joint pain. Behavioural problems are common, especially in children, such as temper tantrums, screaming attacks, sulky behaviour and ultrasensitive personality. Adults may display fatigue, mood swings, anxiety, loss of sexual libido and compulsive behaviour.

The most serious form of allergic reaction is called anaphylactic shock. This is a potentially life-threatening condition involving dangerously lowered blood pressure, collapse and unconsciousness. People known to be at risk of anaphylactic shock often carry an emergency syringe of adrenaline which, if administered promptly, can counteract shock.

ALLERGIES AND ENERGY LEVELS

Research carried out in Iceland in the early 1990s found that fatigue could be directly linked to allergy. In the study, 200 people were tested for a specific and relatively common allergy to a wheat protein and were also tested for iron deficiency (anaemia) and a variety of symptoms including fatigue. The 16 per cent found to have the allergy also had slight deficiencies in iron, although none were diagnosed as anaemic, and the group had complained of fatigue, headaches

and unexplained bouts of diarrhoea to a significantly greater extent than those without the allergy. Researchers concluded that an allergy could cause a number of side effects, including fatigue, which may decrease the quality of life of sufferers without them even knowing it.

A common method of identifying a food allergy is through one of the three types of skin test. Prick testing involves a tiny amount of the possible allergen being introduced into the superficial layer of the skin. In intracutaneous testing a larger dose of the allergen is injected directly into the dermis. It is a more sensitive test, although it is more uncomfortable and less practical than the prick test, and is mostly used as a follow-up. The patch test involves a plaster doused with the allergen that is fixed to the skin and monitored for an allergic response.

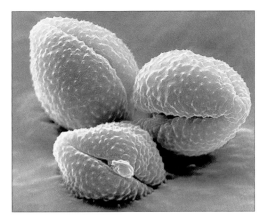

POLLEN
Under the microscope, pollen can be seen to have an aerodynamic shape that helps it to stay airborne. Pollen causes respiratory irritations when it enters the lungs of hayfever sufferers.

65

ENVIRONMENTAL FACTORS

An important aspect of your health is the environment in which you live, work and spend your free time. Healthy, revitalising surroundings can greatly boost your energy.

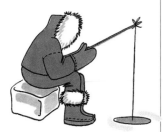

THE TOLLS OF TEMPERATURE
Extreme temperatures lower your energy and ability to work because your body is using much of its energy to adapt to the environment.

A number of different environmental factors can drain your energy without you even being aware of it. The most common problems are associated with the buildings in which we live and work. Creating an atmosphere conducive to energy and good health requires an understanding of the fundamental needs of people. Good, clean air is of great importance, particularly a good supply of fresh air to keep oxygen levels high. Air free from pollutants is also important. Airborne pollutants, such as dust and smoke particles or gas fumes, can all drain energy and can, in the long-run, cause major health risks, especially to the lungs and respiratory system.

Opening windows regularly, if possible, helps to keep air moving and reduces contamination from polluting paints, varnishes,

smoke and dust, which contribute to environmental energy drainage. However, more subtle techniques, such as paying particular attention to furniture positioning and decoration, can boost energy in many directions. The art of feng shui uses the furnishings in a room to enhance and direct energy in a positive way. The techniques are based on traditional Chinese theories of universal energy, or chi, and a system equating the directions of the compass with the different aspects of a person's nature and lifestyle.

Temperature factors

Temperature is another important element as your activity levels are directly affected by the heat and the cold. The body's natural processes work best within a narrow band of temperatures. The best temperature for maximum energy is around 25°C (77°F) – any colder will demand that you use your energy to keep warm, while any warmer will make work more strenuous.

Hot, humid weather is particularly debilitating because the body's main system of losing heat – sweating – requires that moisture evaporates from the surface of the skin, but the high water content of the air makes this more difficult, which can lead to rapid overheating. Of course the effect of external

---

COSMIC ENERGY FORCES: *The Wind*

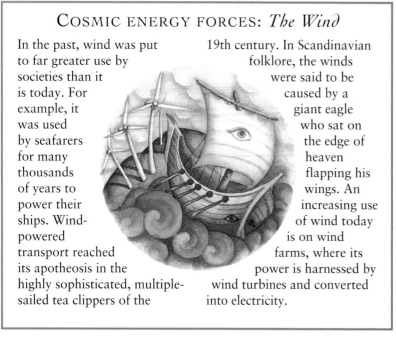

In the past, wind was put to far greater use by societies than it is today. For example, it was used by seafarers for many thousands of years to power their ships. Wind-powered transport reached its apotheosis in the highly sophisticated, multiple-sailed tea clippers of the 19th century. In Scandinavian folklore, the winds were said to be caused by a giant eagle who sat on the edge of heaven flapping his wings. An increasing use of wind today is on wind farms, where its power is harnessed by wind turbines and converted into electricity.

COMPUTER AND TV SCREENS

Watching a VDU screen for long periods of time can be highly stressful, leading to headaches and muscular pains; it is especially tiring for the eyes. Office workers and others who spend long periods in front of a screen are advised to take frequent screen breaks to rest their eyes. You should also exercise your eyes regularly by looking across the room or out of the window and focusing on a distant object. Similar techniques can help to reduce eye strain caused by excessive television viewing. Restricting your viewing hours is often best – get out of the house and do something active.

temperatures can be compounded by other factors. When doing strenuous physical work, for example, your body produces excess heat, which adds to the problem of overheating. Genetic makeup and physical characteristics, such as skin colour, also help to determine how quickly your body adjusts to climate changes.

Noise factors

Unless you wear ear-plugs, you cannot help hearing the noise around you. Excessive or irritating noise can be distracting and stressful, and quickly become physically and emotionally draining. Keeping noise levels down can help to reduce stress. However, sometimes it may be more relaxing to have soothing music, or restful sounds such as ocean waves or countryside noises, playing softly in the background.

LIGHT

Light is a crucial element of life which has an important energising effect on all living things. Getting the lighting right inside buildings can be difficult. Natural daylight is always preferable, but electric lighting is often needed to boost light levels during the day as well as for night-time illumination.

Constant low light levels can affect mood. A widely recognised complaint is low energy and depression caused by lack of sunlight in the winter months, known as seasonal affective disorder (SAD). SAD particularly affects people in countries with very short days in the winter, such as in Scandinavia,

but it is also known in countries with less extreme winters, such as Britain. It is not exactly understood why lack of sunlight has this effect, but the problem can be treated with exposure to bright light screens or by taking regular breaks in a sunnier climate.

There are a number of ways in which to enhance natural light and boost the energising effect of your home. Curtain rails should extend beyond the window so that, when open, the curtains do not cover any part of it, thus allowing in more light. Mirrors can be positioned to reflect the light from windows, enhancing the natural light in a room. Choosing light colours for walls and ceilings will also help to make the most of available light. Skylights can greatly improve the light energies within a room, and in the right situation are relatively easy to fit.

IN THE WORKPLACE

Environmental factors can greatly influence work output, and many industries have found that stress-related problems can be reduced through better control of the work environment. Improving conditions by, for example, altering light, noise, humidity or temperature levels is known to influence physical and mental performance and keep employees happier and less disturbed by external factors. This may be because of the effect of such factors on the hypothalamus, which monitors environmental conditions and alters energy output accordingly.

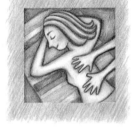

ENERGY BOOST

Treat yourself to a body massage to soothe away the tension in your body. You can find a professional masseur, or ask a friend or family member.

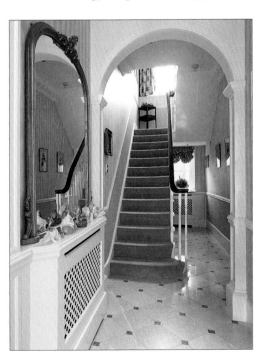

LETTING THE SUNLIGHT INTO YOUR LIFE
Making the most of natural light in your home through windows, mirrors and decoration, can greatly enhance feelings of energy and warmth.

CHRONIC PAIN

Causing constant discomfort and distress, chronic pain drains energy as the body attempts to repair damage, compensate for impaired function, and cope with the pain itself.

The term chronic pain describes pain that is ongoing, lasting for months or even years, as opposed to acute pain which is sudden and temporary. The long-term nature of chronic pain makes it particularly debilitating. One of the main difficulties is the emotional and psychological strain imposed by trying to lead a normal and active life while handicapped by having to cope with constant suffering.

Lack of energy is often compounded by problems caused by trying to compensate for the affected area and lessen the pain. For example, pain in the lower back may cause the sufferer to adopt an unnatural posture in order to take pressure off the problem area. Muscles that would normally be relaxed have to put in extra work and so use up larger amounts of energy. This also puts excess load on neighbouring muscles and joints that may be unused to it, causing further damage and pain in those areas. As a result, the sufferer feels exhausted merely from sitting, walking or standing. People suffering from osteoarthritis in the leg joints may find that a short, slow walk is a major muscle-working exercise, demanding a well-deserved rest afterwards.

CHRONIC HEAD PAIN

Chronic head disorders, including headaches and migraines, cause great stress which is very draining on energy reserves. Headaches are usually caused by tension in the muscles and blood vessels of the scalp and rarely last more than a few hours. They can be triggered by several factors including noise, stress, hunger and fatigue.

Migraines are a particular type of headache that can leave the sufferer bedridden for hours or even days. The throbbing pain of migraines is caused by spasms – the constriction and expansion – of blood vessels in the membranes (meninges) surrounding the brain. They are often triggered by chemicals in food such as citrus fruits, chocolate, cheese and red wine, although stress, heightened emotional states, menstruation and the contraceptive pill are also causal factors.

PAIN IN THE JOINTS

Joint disorders, such as osteoarthritis and rheumatoid arthritis, can cause severe chronic pain. Osteoarthritis is a condition in which the cartilage lining the joints breaks down resulting in movement difficulties. It usually affects the hips, knees and

BOWEN TECHNIQUE

This therapy is reputed to be highly beneficial for many types of physical pain. It incorporates a soft tissue massage technique that works only on the muscles, tendons and ligaments of the body, very gently and with minimal pressure. The treatment can be performed through light clothing, and no oils or special equipment are required. The gentleness of the technique makes it ideal for treating the elderly or very young, or when treatment would otherwise be difficult, perhaps due to a very recent and painful injury.

Regardless of the specific problem being treated, most people respond with a general energy boost, less pain and a better outlook on life. The technique is wonderfully relaxing and can be useful in reducing stress.

The way the technique works has been described by comparing the body to a light switch. The light and the switch may both be working, but if the wires are not connected up properly then the light will not work. Bowen therapy helps to re-establish good connections between the body and brain.

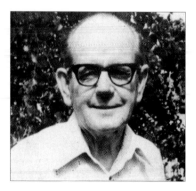

TOM BOWEN
Australian Tom Bowen developed his technique in the 1950s and has since helped over 2000 patients.

spine and is most common in people aged over 60. Rheumatoid arthritis is an autoimmune disorder in which the immune system attacks the joints for no apparent reason. It can occur at any joint in the body, most commonly the hands, wrists, feet and ankles, and may affect people of any age. In some cases food allergies or intolerances aggravate symptoms.

Both forms of arthritis cause pain in the joints, sometimes with swelling and stiffness. In advanced states, sufferers find any movement of the affected joints difficult and very painful, and the extra effort needed for movement drains energy levels.

BACK PAIN

Chronic or sporadic backache is one of the most common pain disorders, affecting an estimated 23 million people in Britain. Back problems are often the result of persistent bad posture; sudden movements, such as twisting, that strain the back muscles; or poor lifting technique, which can damage muscles or vertebrae. Stress is also thought to contribute to back problems as it causes muscular tension which restricts flexibility and increases the risk of muscle strains.

Manipulative therapies, such as osteopathy, chiropractic, physiotherapy and massage therapies, have all been proven to be effective in relieving back pain. General relaxation techniques are also beneficial as they help the muscles to relax and also alleviate stress. People react differently to the various treatments available, however, and sufferers may need to try different kinds until they find the one that is most effective for them.

USING A PAIN DIARY

If you suffer from chronic pain take a little time every day to make some notes about it. This will help you to build up a picture of what triggers your pain, what makes it better, and what makes it worse. Firstly, describe how you feel on that particular day. Try to be as expressive as possible – it does not matter if it sounds silly, just so long as you understand what you mean. Many people use a visual scale to compare how they feel from one day to the next. The scale goes from 0, meaning no pain, to 10, the worst pain experienced.

Make a note of what you ate each day and how it made you feel. This can help you to identify foods that make your condition worse. Note down any activities you undertook as well, and how tired you felt afterwards. This will allow you to draw on knowledge of previous situations before tackling something new. You may find that you are capable of more than you think.

Controlling pain
Researchers have found that you can often reduce pain by actively focusing your attention on a non-painful stimulus. For example, performing mental arithmetic exercises, such as counting backwards by 25 from 1000, or even singing a favourite song can distract your brain from focusing on the pain.

PAIN PATHWAYS

When an excess of any type of stimulus is felt, be it pressure, heat, or cold, the pain receptors under the skin signal to the spinal cord via sensory neurons. The message is sent up the spinal cord to the thalamus, where impulses are sent into the parietal lobes. The individual now becomes aware of the sensation of pain and can assess how best to respond.

PAIN TRANSMISSION
Different types of pain send different chemical messages to the brain, formulating specific responses.

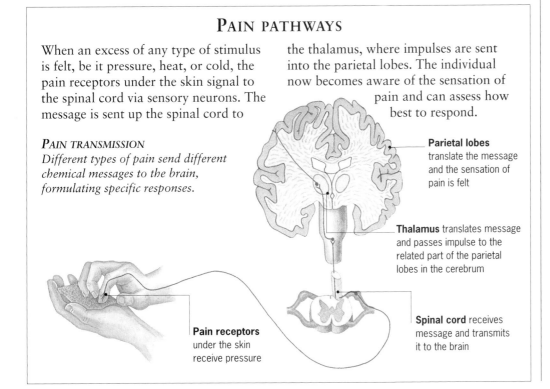

Parietal lobes translate the message and the sensation of pain is felt

Thalamus translates message and passes impulse to the related part of the parietal lobes in the cerebrum

Spinal cord receives message and transmits it to the brain

Pain receptors under the skin receive pressure

Relieving Chronic Pain Fatigue with

Natural Pain Beaters

Living with chronic pain presents a tough challenge to even the most positive of people. Natural pain relievers and careful adjustments to lifestyle can greatly increase your energy levels, allowing you to get more out of life.

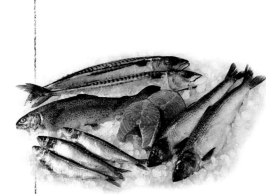

FISH OILS FOR ARTHRITIS
Fish oils are not only mineral and vitamin-packed, they also contain omega-3 fatty acids which are beneficial for arthritis. The best sources are (clockwise from top) herrings, mackerel sardines, trout and salmon (centre). Tinned fish is not as beneficial as many nutrients are lost in the canning process.

Most people suffer from periods of pain in their lives, although these are usually temporary and easily forgotten. However, some people live with ongoing or recurring pain which can eat away at their energy and prevent them from enjoying a full and happy life. Coping with this kind of pain is a two-step process. The first step is to come to terms with the pain and understand what is causing it. The second step is to master the pain. This involves both physical treatments and mental control – you need to think positively and not allow the pain to rule your life. Conventional medicine can help many conditions, although there are some problems which cannot be treated or can only be partially treated. In all circumstances, natural pain remedies and treatments offer useful complementary methods to help you to deal with your pain.

NATURAL THERAPIES

There are various natural therapies that can effectively ease pain and help certain conditions. Working with hands, herbs, water or more complicated equipment, they can help to relax and soothe both body and spirit, allowing you to build up energy and restore well-being.

Touch therapies

There are a number of touch therapies, ranging from a basic massage to the more sophisticated physiotherapy techniques, that can be used to ease pain conditions and aid recovery. Some traditional touch therapies from Asia are becoming quite widespread in this country and can provide a more spiritual approach to pain relief. Tui Na is a massage technique based upon the power of the acupressure points. These are the gateways of the energy channels

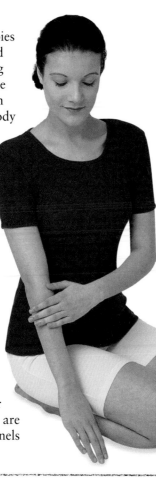

SELF-MASSAGE
You can soothe your body at home with a relaxing self-massage. You don't need to massage your whole body; it can be better to focus on the part that is giving you pain or problems. Acupressure points, held for a few minutes, can be helpful in pain relief.

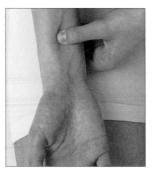

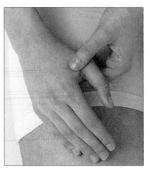

Pericardium 6 is a very powerful point, used for nausea, emotional pain and anxiety. It is particularly good for strengthening the heartbeat. It is located between the two large tendons three finger-widths above the wrist

Large Intestine 4 is one of the most powerful points for calmness and well-being, although it must not be used during pregnancy as it can cause miscarriage. It regulates the body and stimulates the immune system. It is located at the base of the V formed between the thumb and index finger

that pass through the body; by pressing the points, energy flow can be improved, promoting better health, vitality and balance. Other Eastern touch therapies that work on energy levels in a similar way include shiatsu and Jin Shin, which originate from Japan.

Reiki involves the passing of energy from a healer to a patient by simply placing the hands on the body and concentrating on the transfer.

Thai massage is vigorous, with the therapist bending and manipulating the patient through a number of movements and positions. Other manipulative therapies include osteopathy, chiropractic and physiotherapy. They are often well-established within the medical framework, sometimes attached to hospitals or doctors' clinics. Osteopathy and chiropractic both aim to restore the proper alignment of the body, particularly the back, in order to rebalance the body and restore it to health. Physiotherapy uses a number of techniques, including ultrasound and hydrotherapy, to promote tissue repair and proper body functioning.

Dietary considerations

A balanced diet with a wide variety of foods and a large proportion of fresh fruit and vegetables can help to alleviate many conditions and prevent the onset or worsening of a number of problems. Make sure that you are getting all the essential minerals and vitamins (see Chapter 4), and take supplements in the form of tablets if you are not certain that you are obtaining all that you need from your food. Avoid refined sugar which can unbalance energy levels, and cut down on fats as they tend to aggravate health problems; saturated fats in particular can lead to cardiovascular disorders.

Try to keep your weight within normal limits. Being either overweight or underweight will aggravate most medical conditions, and obesity can lead to severe energy problems that will hinder recovery.

Positive thinking

Try to perceive your body as a whole, encompassing both the pain and the parts that function and work well, and try to put the pain into context. Remember that you are an energised being with the power to achieve what you want. Becoming a slave to pain is all too easy – shun it by taking control of your life and not letting it get you down. A good night's sleep, without the use of sleeping pills or drugs, will always help you to recover your energy levels and leave you feeling refreshed.

NATURAL PAINKILLERS

Herbal remedies have been used for thousands of years to combat pain. Some of the more tried-and-tested natural pain remedies are listed below, but be sure to check with your doctor if you have a serious complaint.

PROBLEM	HERBAL REMEDY	PREPARATION
Stomach ulcers	Liquorice	Drink herbal infusion
Indigestion	Meadowsweet, Marshmallow, Peppermint, Fennel	Drink herbal infusion or eat as sweets
Nausea	Ginger, Black horehound	Drink herbal infusion
Constipation	Yellow dock	Drink herbal infusion
Diarrhoea	Agrimony	Drink herbal infusion
Breathing problems	Thyme, Eucalyptus	Breathe in infusion
Period pains	Lady's mantle, Shepherd's purse	Drink herbal infusion
Throat problems	Sage	Drink herbal infusion
Headache	Vervain	Place cold compress of infusion on neck
Muscle damage	Vulneraries, Camomile	Drink herbal infusion
Rheumatic pain	Rosemary, Eucalyptus, Clove	Drink herbal infusion
Muscle pain	St John's wort, Lavender	Apply onto skin
Arthritis	Rosemary, Ginger, Cloves	Bathe or apply onto skin

Thyme prepared in a herbal tea is good for breathing problems

Rosemary can be used in creams and massage oils for arthritis

Sage can be drunk as a tea for throat problems

Cloves can be made into a tea to help rheumatic pain

DIETS THAT DRAIN ENERGY

Food and drink are the source of your basic energy requirements. If you are not eating the correct balance of energy and nutrients, you may find yourself feeling lethargic and lacking in vitality.

EMPTY CALORIES
Fruit and vegetables have far more nutrients per calorie than many over-refined fast foods.

Food and drink provide your body with the wealth of nutrients and fuels that are necessary to keep you alive and functioning properly. The role that many minerals, vitamins and other nutrients play in keeping us healthy and in preventing disease is still not fully understood, and there is controversy over the amounts of certain nutrients that you need for optimum health. However, there are some basic guidelines that you should follow to ensure that your diet is providing the energy you need.

NUTRITIONAL DEFICIENCY
Certain basic nutrients are necessary for the proper functioning of the body and any deficiency will result in a loss of energy, as well as other symptoms. The combination of nutrients that a body needs to function forms a complex pattern of chemical reactions and interactions. A varied diet is vital to ensure your body receives all the nutrients it needs in the right combination to achieve maximum energy output and optimum functioning. In some situations, however, you may need to increase your intake of certain nutrients in order to boost your energy levels – when recovering from an illness, for example. Disorders that

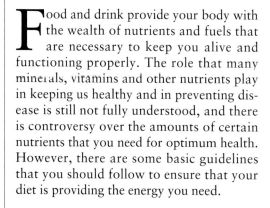

cause repeated vomiting or diarrhoea can quickly deplete the body of vital trace elements and will also prevent your body from extracting all the nourishment available in your food. As a result you may need to increase your intake of vitamins and minerals to compensate. Vomiting and diarrhoea can also cause serious dehydration, so it is important to increase your fluid intake to replace what has been lost.

Many women suffer iron deficiency anaemia because large amounts of this mineral, found particularly in red blood cells, can be lost during menstruation. Anaemia commonly affects energy levels, leading to chronic fatigue. Diets that are low in magnesium, zinc, vitamin B_1 (thiamine) and B_{12} can also lead to reduced energy levels. More information about these nutrients and the other energy-linked vitamins and minerals can be found in Chapter 4, including details about the best food sources.

DIETING AND WEIGHT CONTROL
Fatigue is a common problem for people who are trying to lose weight, particularly if they are not following a properly balanced diet plan set by a qualified nutritionist. Problems mainly arise when the dieter

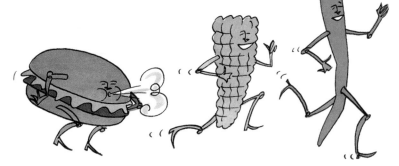

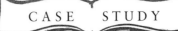

The Caffeine Addict

Taking stimulants such as caffeine to help you to wake up in the morning can lead to a vicious circle of exhaustion and a growing need for more caffeine, compounding the situation and resulting in chronic fatigue. Facing your problems and dealing with stress through relaxation, a healthy diet and a regular sleeping pattern can help you to rebalance your natural energy levels.

Damien is a newspaper reporter in his late 20s. He has recently been promoted and has found it difficult to keep up with his new workload. This is compounded by an active social life, involving heavy drinking with friends most evenings. In order to get through his work, he has been getting into the office earlier in the morning and using large doses of strong coffee to boost his energy. He has felt himself becoming increasingly exhausted, however, and is depending more and more on caffeine to keep awake. He can see that a vicious circle of tiredness and coffee addiction is starting to adversely affect his whole life. A concerned colleague has advised him to do something before he has a nervous collapse.

WHAT SHOULD DAMIEN DO?

Damien needs to regain control over his work and life. Although initially sceptical, he went to see a traditional Chinese medical practitioner. The practitioner explained how Damien's excessive use of caffeine was actually making his exhaustion worse in the long run. He recommended that Damien revise his drinking and social habits and forgo coffee. Cutting out caffeine would be difficult at first but, in the long run, it would allow Damien's natural energy levels to improve. The practitioner recommended a programme of acupuncture and herbal treatment to help Damien to overcome his caffeine addiction and counter the stress factors in his life.

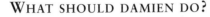

Action Plan

HEALTH
Cut down on alcohol consumption to improve sleep. Get into the habit of going to bed and getting up at regular times.

DIET
Cut down on caffeine intake and resist the urge to take a quick energy boost – it will sap energy in the long run and leave you needing more.

LIFESTYLE
Restrict drinking with friends to the weekends and keep weekdays free for work, relaxation and good sleep. Give up smoking.

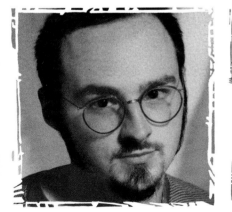

HEALTH
Irregular sleeping patterns and too much alcohol make large demands on energy levels.

DIET
Drinking too much coffee can boost energy temporarily but leads to fatigue in the long term.

LIFESTYLE
Keeping up a hectic social life can leave you lacking vitality for work.

HOW THINGS TURNED OUT FOR DAMIEN

At first, Damien very much missed both his coffee and his regular nights out, although the acupuncture helped him to relax and overcome his coffee cravings. After a few weeks, he felt his energy levels start to improve. Soon he was mentally and physically alert throughout the day at work. He has joined a gym and his twice-weekly work-outs have helped his energy levels even more – and he really looks forward to his nights out at weekends.

wants to lose weight quickly, for a wedding for example, and cuts down food intake severely in a crash diet.

Generally, a crash diet does not provide enough readily available energy for the body's basic requirements and often lacks vital vitamins and minerals. In crash diets, the available energy stores are used quickly, leaving only the long-term fat stores to fuel the body. These are not so readily converted into energy and so the dieter will end up feeling tired and lacking in vitality. As well as a loss of energy, this can lead to weakness, lethargy, headaches, digestive upsets and mental disorders such as depression. The body's basal metabolic rate also slows in an emergency reaction to the reduced food intake. This slows the rate at which stored fat is used and so makes the diet less effective as a weight-loss programme.

The body needs a certain level of energy in order to burn up fat stores. A nutritionist or dietitian will take this into account when planning a diet for you, as well as ensuring that your meals have adequate levels of vitamins and minerals. A properly planned weight-loss diet is both healthier and more efficient than a crash diet.

Long-term restrictive diets can also be detrimental to energy levels unless they are carefully monitored. Vegetarians, and more particularly vegans who do not eat any animal products at all, can enjoy perfect health but need to take care to eat properly. People with eating disorders such as anorexia nervosa and bulimia limit their food intake drastically, in the first case by self-imposed starvation, and in the second by forced

EXTRA HEALTHY DIETS
The Mediterranean diet is considered to be one of the world's healthiest. The fresh fruit and vegetables, herbs and fresh seafood contribute greatly to the diet's nutritional value. Tasty olive oil is used as a healthy and nourishing cooking medium. Red wine is used in cooking and drunk with the meal, aiding digestion and relaxation – one of the best prescriptions for good health.

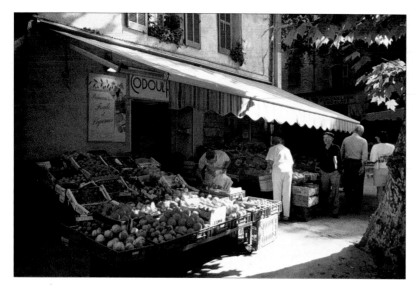

Origins

The condition of anaemia was first identified by a German physician, Dr Johannes Lange, who wrote a paper in 1554 entitled 'Concerning the Disease of the Virgins'. In the paper he describes the weakness and fatigue suffered by young women, characterised by shortness of breath and poor appetite. Lange named the condition 'chlorosis' because the sufferer's complexion was so pale that it was almost green.

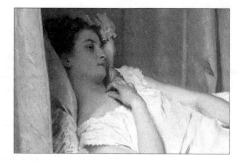

CHLOROSIS
This anaemic condition is associated with young women, romantically depicted through history as weak and fainting.

vomiting or excessive use of laxatives. This leads to greatly reduced energy levels and potentially long-term health disorders.

OVERWEIGHT AND OBESITY
Calories that are consumed but not converted into energy for powering basic bodily processes or physical activities will be stored as adipose tissue, a form of fat. Excess storage of fat leads to being overweight, which can affect energy levels in several ways. The strain of carrying excess weight makes people tire faster and they tend to become less mobile as a result. This reduces the amount of energy that is burned up, so that even more of the calorie intake is stored as fat.

Excess fat can lead to serious health problems, such as raised blood pressure which puts excess strain on the heart and blood vessels. This leads to breathlessness, fatigue, reduced mobility and increased weight-gain, causing a downward spiral that can result in serious weight problems and obesity.

An estimated 30 per cent of the UK population is overweight, with five per cent being obese, in other words extremely overweight.

Obesity is defined by the British Medical Association as being 'more than 20 per cent over your maximum desirable weight'. It affects a person in much the same way as being overweight, but in a more severe form. In addition to the physical problems caused by being overweight, obesity often carries a social stigma which can deter sufferers from leaving their homes, leading to a further lack of mobility and increased fat deposition. Chronic lack of exercise can exacerbate health problems further and increase the build-up of unused fat stores. Increased isolation is another common result which can lead to mental problems such as depression.

Appetite and behaviour

There has been much research establishing links between overweight, overeating and the feeling of being satiated – being satisfied with the amount of food that you have eaten. It has been shown to be a very complex issue, involving metabolism, genetic make-up, and emotional and psychological factors, as well as the type and amount of food. Research with animals suggests that if food is rich in protein and highly palatable then more than normal will be eaten.

Emotional factors have also been found to make a marked difference to appetite. For example, appetite tends to increase during times of stress, anxiety and depression, whereas maintaining a relaxed, calm mood tends to stabilise or decrease appetite.

Obesity has been called a disease of food abuse and can sometimes be tackled by checking the impulse for binge eating. There are practical tips you can follow to avoid excess eating. They include drinking plenty of water before and during meals to help fill you up, putting meals on smaller plates so you are not tempted to serve yourself too much, chewing more slowly and pausing longer between mouthfuls to allow the food time to go down, avoiding snacks between meals, and filling up with fresh fruit and vegetables. It can also help to consume most of your calories during the day and only have a light meal in the evening.

It is important to realise that often people eat not just because they are hungry but also because of social situations. For example, a considerable amount of overeating is related to the tradition of dining out – either for business reasons or with friends – where multiple courses are eaten out of custom rather than hunger. Business lunches are a particularly difficult problem since it is considered bad manners to opt out of, say, having a starter. Many people find themselves eating more when they start living with someone else with different needs. Women particularly fall into this trap because their needs are usually less than men's, although they often eat a similar amount.

ENERGY BOOST

A 200 ml glass of half-fat milk contains 7 g of protein, 10 g of carbohydrate and 30 per cent of your daily recommended calcium intake – and only 100 kcals.

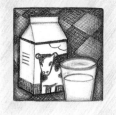

YIN AND YANG FOODS

Traditional Chinese medicine promotes a balance between yin, the female force, and yang, the male force. Diet plays a major role in balancing your energies, particularly by rebalancing overactive energies with the opposite energy foods.

Yang foods include meat and fish, alcohol, cooked vegetables, mango, nuts and beans

Yin foods include soft fruit, bamboo shoots, watermelon, honey, chillis, salad and lemons

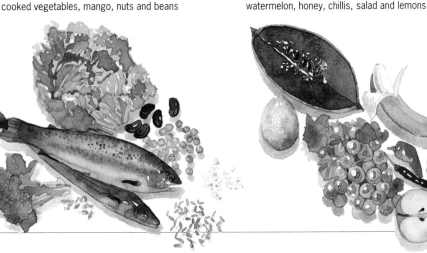

Daytime Drowsiness

One of the most common signs of fatigue is drowsiness during the day, often occurring in episodes in the afternoon and early evening. There are a number of ways to avoid or curb daytime drowsiness.

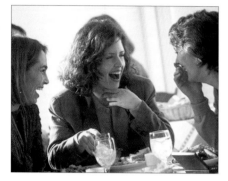

HAVE SOME FUN
Balancing work with fun can help to keep your motivation up. Taking on a variety of tasks, rather than plodding away at one lengthy task, can also help you to stay awake and active.

Feelings of drowsiness can affect people in different ways; some feel drained all day, whereas others find themselves dropping into a light sleep after a meal. Whichever way it affects you, daytime drowsiness can seriously disrupt your ability to get on with normal life.

There are many factors that can cause daytime drowsiness, including poor sleep at night, a poor diet, or a more serious condition or illness. It is important initially to try to locate the cause of the drowsiness. This chapter, as well as Chapter 6, describes and explains some of the common problems and conditions associated with fatigue. If you think that you may be suffering from a more serious illness, you must see your doctor. You should also seek the advice of a doctor if your drowsiness continues after following the suggestions below and opposite.

ORGANISING YOUR LIFE TO PREVENT DROWSINESS

You can help your energy problems by planning your life to fit in with them. If you realise that your body is telling you to slow down and that you may be trying to fit too much into your day, you are well on the way to some practical solutions to your daytime drowsiness. The key to a healthy life is to listen to your body and its needs. When your body tells you that it is tired, you should take a rest and try to work out the factors that are making you tired so that you can avoid them in the future.

STRETCHING
If you find yourself getting sleepy you may find that a good stretch gets your blood flowing. This exercise helps the blood flow to your head, revitalising your mind.

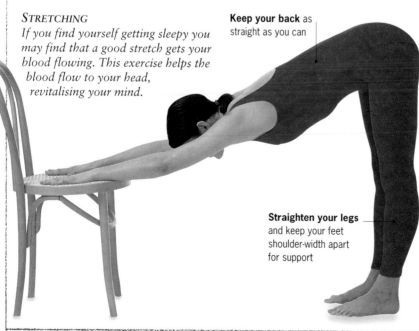

Keep your back as straight as you can

Straighten your legs and keep your feet shoulder-width apart for support

ENERGISING TIPS

Taking time to plan your life can help you to find energy when you need it.

▶ *Consider your energy priorities. Make a list of all the things that you need to do and then list them in priority. If you do not have the energy to do everything, make sure that the ones that get left out are those at the bottom, and are carried forward to the next list.*

▶ *Do not waste your energy on worrying. People often lose sleep and suffer from tiredness following an anxious period. Try not to let yourself be drawn in. Worrying about something will not make the problem better.*

▶ *Take a brisk walk to get some fresh air into your lungs and increase your heartbeat. This will speed the flow of blood around your body, enabling you to think, move and react faster. A 10-minute walk is all that is needed.*

DRINKS AND YOUR ENERGY LEVELS

Many people ignore the health aspects of drinks, although they can play a major part in providing energy – for example, milk shakes and juices – or in reducing it, as fizzy drinks and alcoholic drinks can. The body needs 1.5 litres (2.6 pints) of fluid every day – make sure you keep yourself topped up.

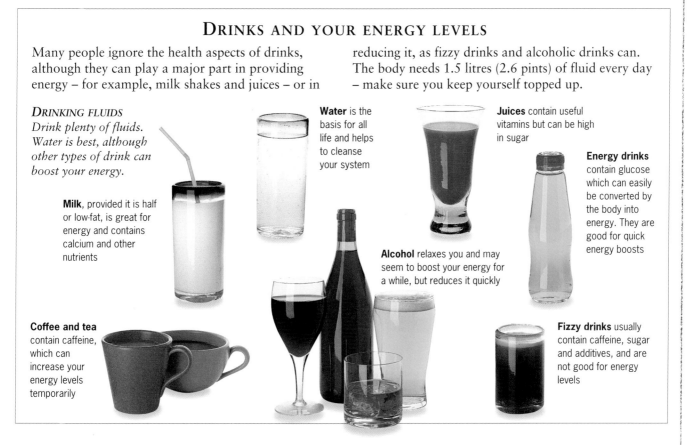

DRINKING FLUIDS
Drink plenty of fluids. Water is best, although other types of drink can boost your energy.

Milk, provided it is half or low-fat, is great for energy and contains calcium and other nutrients

Coffee and tea contain caffeine, which can increase your energy levels temporarily

Water is the basis for all life and helps to cleanse your system

Alcohol relaxes you and may seem to boost your energy for a while, but reduces it quickly

Juices contain useful vitamins but can be high in sugar

Energy drinks contain glucose which can easily be converted by the body into energy. They are good for quick energy boosts

Fizzy drinks usually contain caffeine, sugar and additives, and are not good for energy levels

DIETARY ADVICE

Keeping your diet healthy and well balanced will help you to tackle daytime drowsiness. Make a note of any times in the day when you feel sleepy, then plan to counteract the tiredness with an energy-giving snack or drink.

▶ *Eat smaller meals more frequently throughout the day. Many people feel tired and sleepy after a heavy meal, whereas after eating a light meal your energy level will temporarily rise.*

▶ *Do not eat heavy meals as your energy will be spent in digesting the food. This is often the reason that people fall asleep after a heavy lunch.*

▶ *Make carbohydrates and fresh fruit and vegetables the main constituents of your diet. Carbohydrates are a long-lasting energy source, and fresh fruit and vegetables should provide you with the nutrients and fibre that you need.*

▶ *Avoid sugary snacks and foods – they may give you a quick energy fix but this will soon wear off, leaving you more tired than before.*

▶ *Drink a cup of tea or coffee. Researchers in Massachusetts have found that the caffeine in a cup of coffee can give you an energy boost that lasts for up to six hours. However, you should limit your intake to three cups a day – more than this can chronically exhaust you.*

ENERGY SNACKS
You can easily boost your energy through the day by having a quick snack. Avoid snacks that contain processed sugar and fat, and focus on those high in carbohydrates and nutrients.

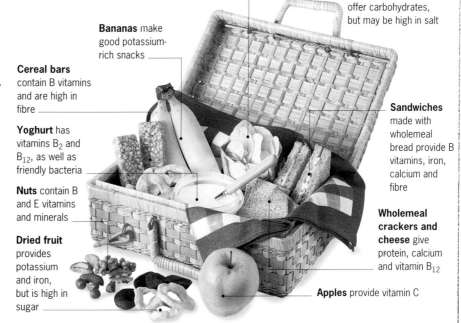

Cereal bars contain B vitamins and are high in fibre

Yoghurt has vitamins B_2 and B_{12}, as well as friendly bacteria

Nuts contain B and E vitamins and minerals

Dried fruit provides potassium and iron, but is high in sugar

Bananas make good potassium-rich snacks

Low-fat potato crisps offer carbohydrates, but may be high in salt

Sandwiches made with wholemeal bread provide B vitamins, iron, calcium and fibre

Wholemeal crackers and cheese give protein, calcium and vitamin B_{12}

Apples provide vitamin C

DRUGS THAT DRAIN ENERGY

Drugs affect the way you function and can alter energy levels in different ways, for example, through their action on brain cells, or by altering your hormone levels and chemical make-up.

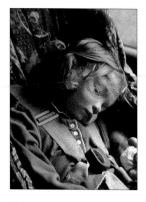

FATIGUE FACTOR
Travel sickness pills, often given to children, can cause drowsiness and loss of energy.

Medicines, either prescription drugs or over-the-counter remedies, are an integral part of the way we deal with illness and health maintenance today. However, the way that drugs act on the body is often poorly understood and the picture is even more unclear when their effect in combination with other drugs or common foodstuffs is taken into account. Small chemical changes and emotional disturbances caused by drugs can lead to a chain reaction that affects energy levels.

PRESCRIPTION DRUGS

A large number of prescription drugs can make you feel tired and lethargic, often because of their effect on neurotransmitters

in the brain. This effect may be even more marked when a drug is taken in combination with some over-the-counter preparations, alcohol or foods such as cheese or chocolate. For this reason, it is important to ask your doctor about possible side effects and check whether certain foods, alcohol or other drugs may cause complications when taking the medication.

Some antidepressants trigger the release of chemicals in the brain that stimulate nerve activity, often leading to feelings of fatigue, lethargy and drowsiness. Similarly, some antipsychotics, used to alleviate severe anxiety and other problematic mental states, can cause lethargy and drowsiness. This is because they work by blocking the action of dopamine, a natural chemical in the brain that stimulates nerve action.

Antiepileptic drugs inhibit electrical activity within the brain to prevent seizures, with the effect of reduced mental alertness. Some drugs used to lower blood pressure can also cause dizziness and fainting. Antivomiting drugs reduce nerve activity at the base of the brain to suppress the vomiting reflex, causing drowsiness and lethargy.

OVER-THE-COUNTER DRUGS

Many drugs that you can buy at chemists have side effects that can greatly influence your energy levels. You must read the instructions carefully and plan to rest after ingestion.

DRUG	POSSIBLE SIDE EFFECTS
Paracetamol	Can cause liver problems. Easy to overdose – do not exceed 4000 mg (about 8 tablets) in 24 hours
Aspirin	Gastric irritation, stomach problems
Ibuprofen	Confusion and lethargy, indigestion
Codeine	Confusion, concentration loss, constipation, addictive
Diclofenac	Lethargy, dizziness, stomach problems
Naproxen	Confusion, loss of concentration, lethargy, stomach problems
D-proxyphene	Sedation, constipation, nausea, slightly addictive
Morphine	Sedation, constipation, addictive

ANTIDEPRESSANTS

Used to lift mood, antidepressants such as Prozac increase the neurotransmitter serotonin in the brain, speeding the transport of information around the brain. This helps to lift people out of their depression, allowing them to take a more detached approach to problems and to resolve anxieties. It can cause lack of concentration and tiredness, although the positive feelings usually counteract any bad effects. The drug takes four to six weeks to work and the wait can debilitate the sufferer severely. Likewise, coming off the drug can be difficult as the body may have stopped producing the normal levels of serotonin naturally. This often leads to more depression and an inability to function properly.

Sleeping pills and tranquillisers are no longer prescribed liberally following the realisation that they suppress the normal sleeping patterns necessary for good physical and mental health. They can also be highly addictive, leading to tolerance and dependency and an inability to sleep properly without the drug.

Drugs and food interactions

Some common foods, especially cheese, wine, grapefruit and tea, can interact with prescription drugs and either block or intensify their effects. Cheese and wine contain monoamines which have a similar chemical structure to some amphetamine drugs and when mixed with other drugs may cause migraines, nightmares, hallucinations and raised blood pressure. It is the monoamines in cheese that are thought to cause nightmares in some people.

Grapefruit reduces the effect of an enzyme in the small intestine which breaks down medicines, increasing the amount that is absorbed by the body. Those taking drugs for hayfever and heart disorders are warned not to eat grapefruit, and some research suggests that women taking the contraceptive pill should also avoid eating the fruit, although this remains contentious.

Tea contains substances that can reduce the effect of some vitamin supplements. It is advisable to allow a gap of at least an hour following a meal or after taking supplements before drinking tea to ensure the proper absorption of vitamins.

OVER-THE-COUNTER DRUGS

Many over-the-counter drugs can alter your energy levels, making you tired, lethargic and unable to concentrate, although remedies often also include caffeine or other stimulants to counteract this effect. Cold remedies in particular often contain drugs such as antihistamines which are used to dry up a runny nose. They can cause drowsiness, fatigue and loss of concentration and daytime use should be avoided.

Paracetamol is the most popular painkiller in Britain and has few side effects; it is also an antipyretic (reduces high temperature). It does not alter energy levels, but the risk of accidental overdose is high, so you must take care to avoid taking different medications that include paracetamol. Aspirin is another popular painkiller and antipyretic and, unlike paracetamol, can alleviate inflammation. It can cause stomach bleeding if taken for long periods, however, and so is unsuitable for those suffering from gastrointestinal disorders. It is not recommended for those with asthma or children under 12, except on a doctor's advice.

THE CONTRACEPTIVE PILL

Although many women enjoy the positive benefits of the contraceptive pill, some find that it drains their energy levels. The contraceptive pill works by altering hormone levels in the body to mimic those of pregnancy, and many of the side effects are similar to the symptoms experienced during early pregnancy, including tiredness. If you think that the pill may be causing energy problems, you may prefer to take the progesterone-only pill which has fewer side effects, although it is slightly less reliable.

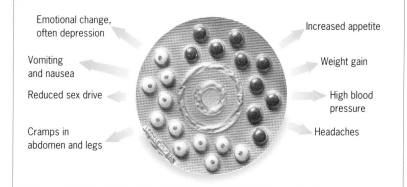

Emotional change, often depression

Vomiting and nausea

Reduced sex drive

Cramps in abdomen and legs

Increased appetite

Weight gain

High blood pressure

Headaches

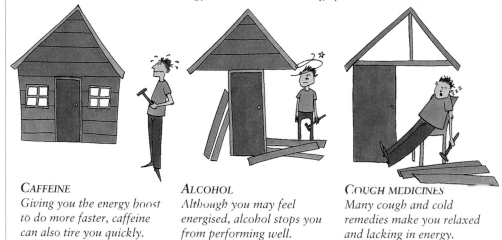

DRUGS AND COMPETENCE

Many commonly taken drugs can greatly affect your ability and motivation to work. The benefits from these drugs are widely utilised, such as the energy boost from caffeine and the relaxing effect of alcohol. However, if you have a job to do, you should consider the side effects of the drugs you intend to take.

CAFFEINE
Giving you the energy boost to do more faster, caffeine can also tire you quickly.

ALCOHOL
Although you may feel energised, alcohol stops you from performing well.

COUGH MEDICINES
Many cough and cold remedies make you relaxed and lacking in energy.

Ibuprofen is a painkiller and anti-inflammatory with fewer side effects than aspirin. It is particularly useful for period pains and rheumatoid arthritis. In susceptible individuals, it can cause lethargy, nausea and other digestive disorders. Codeine is a very effective narcotic painkiller derived from the opium poppy and it is used in combination with other painkillers. It may make you drowsy, so don't plan anything strenuous.

NICOTINE
Nicotine is a stimulant found in the tobacco plant and is usually taken through smoking the tobacco leaves. The predominant effects are on the autonomic nervous system which controls the automatic, involuntary body functions, such as heart rate and breathing. The drug works in different ways from person to person. Someone not used to nicotine will experience a lowering of the heart rate, whereas a nicotine addict will have an increased heartbeat and raised blood pressure. Nicotine also stimulates the central nervous system, increasing alertness and improving concentration, but it is also addictive and users need progressively larger amounts to stimulate their system.

ALCOHOL
Alcohol depresses the central nervous system, decreasing the activity of the brain and spinal cord and therefore reducing anxiety, tension and inhibitions. It is used widely throughout most of the world for its relaxing qualities, and in small quantities it may help to relieve stress. However, performance rapidly deteriorates with increased alcohol intake, as it impairs both mental and physical functions. It has a slight stimulant effect that can delay the onset of fatigue for a while, but continued drinking causes sleepiness and even unconsciousness. The following day you may find yourself lacking in concentration and dehydrated.

STEROID DRUGS
Anabolic steroids are sometimes taken to increase muscle size in body builders and athletes, increasing energy potential. They are derived from the male hormone testosterone and can cause aggression and a number of side effects influencing the sexual functioning and characteristics of a person.

RECREATIONAL DRUGS
Some people take 'recreational' drugs to change their mood and energy levels. Some of these drugs are also used in a psychiatric framework to study the workings of the human mind and to help individuals to express their anxieties and deeper emotional worries. However, most are not conducive in the long term to good physical and psychological health, and they often entail de-energising withdrawal symptoms.

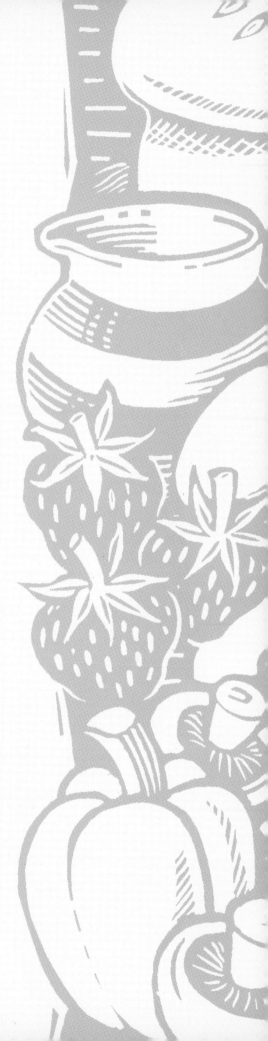

CHAPTER 4

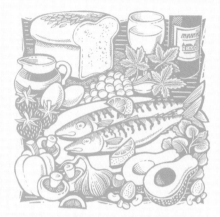

EATING FOR ENERGY

Recent studies have clearly shown the important role that diet plays in preventing disease and illness. If you understand the essential components of healthy eating, as well as the role that particular nutrients have in energy production, you can eat to optimise your health and energy.

THE COMPONENTS OF HEALTHY EATING

Energy comes direct from the food that you eat, so if you understand the basic elements of healthy eating, improved well-being and vitality will be within your grasp.

Energy is needed by the human body to function and to be active. The body gets this energy from the major components of food which are carbohydrate, fat and protein, and alcohol can also be used. This energy is measured in kilocalories, more commonly referred to as calories.

The human body produces energy in much the same way as a railway engine – fuel is used to feed a process that releases energy as a product. The essential difference between the human body and a railway engine is that in the body the energy is released gradually by a series of steps, each carefully controlled by enzymes and hormones. This energy can then be used by the body for movement and other vital processes. Unfortunately, the human body is not as efficient as the railway engine, and a large amount of energy is lost as heat.

The body obtains energy or calories from the three main nutrients. Carbohydrates provide energy for immediate use, or can be

YOUR DAILY DIET

For the best of health and vitality, a balanced diet consisting mostly of complex carbohydrates, fruit and vegetables is advised. Cutting fats and sugars down to a portion of your daily food intake, and keeping dairy products to a minimum, will also be of benefit.

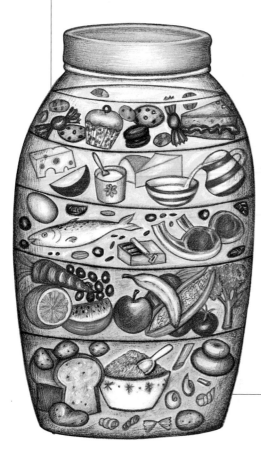

BASIC DIET
A balanced diet consists of a variety of foods consumed in different quantities.

Foods containing fat and sugar
should be kept to a minimum. Snacks often contain surprisingly large amounts of unhealthy saturated fats

Milk and dairy foods
should be eaten in moderation. Choose lower-fat alternatives

Meat, fish and other protein foods
should be eaten in moderate amounts. If you are vegetarian include pulses, nuts and seeds in your diet

Fruit and vegetables
should provide a good proportion of your diet. The minimum goal is five portions a day, not including potatoes

Grains, bread, pasta and potatoes
should provide the bulk of your diet. If you are dieting, cut out fat and sugar, not grains and carbohydrates

THREE DIET RULES

The World Health Organization (WHO) recommends three rules to help to reduce the death toll from the two main killers of the late 20th century – heart disease and cancer.

▶ *Half of your food intake should consist of starchy, complex carbohydrates such as bread, pasta, rice, potatoes. Brown, wholegrain or wholemeal versions have the most nutrients. For variety try other forms of grains like polenta, couscous, or millet and quinoa.*

▶ *Eat at least five portions of fruit and vegetables each day. Choose a wide variety of fresh, frozen and dried forms.*

▶ *Cut saturated fat, found mostly in meats and dairy products, to a minimum. By eating more fruit, vegetables, low-fat and starchy fibre-rich foods it is easy to achieve this third rule.*

EAT YOUR GREENS

The health benefits derived from eating plenty of fruit and vegetables can be seen by comparing dietary intake to rates of heart disease throughout Western Europe.

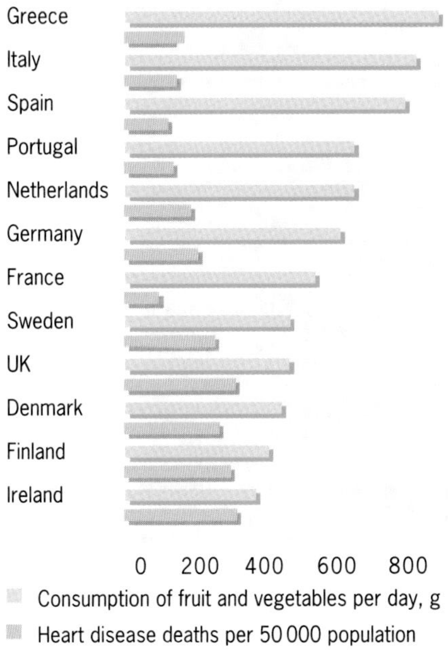

Greece		
Italy		
Spain		
Portugal		
Netherlands		
Germany		
France		
Sweden		
UK		
Denmark		
Finland		
Ireland		

0   200   400   600   800

Consumption of fruit and vegetables per day, g

Heart disease deaths per 50 000 population

PREVENTING HEART DISEASE
Eating five portions of fruit and vegetables every day reduces the risk of heart disease by an estimated 20 per cent.

health. Thinking about the balance of the major food groups makes it easier to control the number of calories that you consume. If you are trying to lose weight, aim to get most of your calories from nutrient-dense foods.

CARBOHYDRATES

These are the main sources of energy in almost all diets worldwide. The term carbohydrate includes both simple sugars and starch. Starches are complex structures composed of interlinked sugar molecules. In the digestive tract, digestive enzymes break down these linked sugar molecules into their constituent single sugars so that they can be absorbed into the bloodstream. The most important sugar to the body is glucose. The body's metabolism and energy systems have a high demand for glucose, and a low level of glucose in the blood results in such a disturbance in brain functioning that, in extreme cases, it can eventually lead to collapse, coma and death.

Historically our ancestors ate considerably more complex carbohydrates and it is only since the middle of the 19th century that our intake of refined carbohydrates, particularly sucrose (ordinary table sugar), has significantly increased.

Several hormones are involved in the control of carbohydrate metabolism, in particular insulin, adrenaline and glucagon. These all work together to maintain a steady blood sugar level (or blood glucose level). The major function of glucose in the body is to produce energy. When there is an excess of glucose in the diet, the extra is stored as glycogen in the liver.

If a person stops eating altogether, the glycogen store in the liver will last for 24 to 48 hours. After that, more glucose has to be produced by converting body fat stores. The glycogen stores are mobilised by adrenaline and glucagon and, therefore, these hormones are directly responsible for raising the blood sugar level.

For glucose to be utilised by the body for energy, it has to cross from the blood into the cell, which requires insulin. Therefore, insulin lowers the blood sugar by helping it to transfer into the cells where it is needed.

A diabetic suffers from a shortage of insulin resulting in the blood sugar level becoming too

stored in the liver as glycogen. Any excess will be converted to fat for storage. Fats also provide energy, but in a more concentrated form than carbohydrates and, again, any excess will be stored as body fat. Proteins provide amino acids, the building blocks of growth and repair. They can also be converted into glycogen for energy.

Minerals and vitamins are also vital. They are used in growth and repair and are involved in regulating body processes through hormones and enzymes. Very few foods contain only one nutrient. Most are complex mixtures of the main nutrients (macro nutrients) with small amounts of vitamins and minerals (micro nutrients).

MACRO AND MICRO NUTRIENTS

Variety not only makes eating more interesting, but also helps to make sure that you get a balance of the different nutrients. Getting this balance right is essential for good

GLUCOSE
Every carbohydrate is broken down into monosaccharides, such as glucose (pictured below), which consists of a hexagonal molecular arrangement of carbon (blue), oxygen (orange) and hydrogen (yellow).

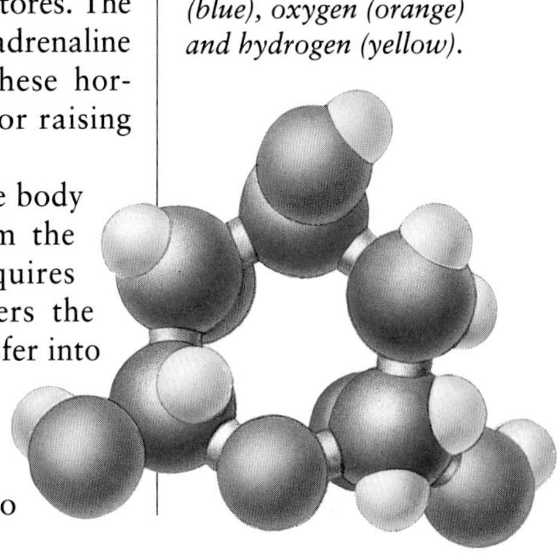

83

THE KREBS CYCLE AND ENERGY PRODUCTION

Inside each cell in the body is a number of small energy factories called mitochondria. Within each of these a reaction takes place whereby a chemical (ATP) splits and creates energy. By splitting, the chemical character of the ATP changes and it becomes ADP. The chemical is restored back to ATP with the use of fuel from glucose and other nutrients. It then splits again, repeating the cycle.

1 The Krebs cycle is a complicated process that combines glucose and other fuels to create phosphate molecules, which are the source of energy production.

2 The phosphate molecule from the Krebs cycle joins the two phosphate molecules from the ADP (adenosine diphosphate) to form energy-producing ATP (adenosine triphosphate).

3 The restored ATP splits, releasing energy and losing a phosphate molecule, thus becoming ADP. The process also uses oxygen and produces carbon dioxide as a by-product, which is expelled from the lungs.

Carbon dioxide

Krebs cycle produces phosphate

Glucose and other fuels

4 The ADP stays in this state until another phosphate molecule provided by the Krebs cycle becomes available.

ATP

ADP

Energy

ADP

P **Phosphate groups**

high with a corresponding shortage of glucose in the cells, leaving the sufferer feeling weak and fatigued (see page 92).

FATS

There are many different kinds of fat, some of which are beneficial, but most should be avoided as they are generally bad for your health and can lead to weight gain.

The bad fats that should be avoided are the saturated fats, found mostly in meats and dairy products. Saturated fats become hard in cool temperatures and can stubbornly remain in arteries and the heart, causing poor heart and artery functioning.

Monounsaturated and polyunsaturated fats are those that remain liquid in cool temperatures, such as vegetable and fish oils. There is evidence from the wide use of olive oil in southern Europe that these oils provide benefits to health, although too much will make you gain weight.

Fish oils are good for you. They are high in fatty acids crucial for proper body functioning. It has been suggested that you should try to eat oily fish, such as tuna, salmon or sardines, at least twice a week. The fatty acids can also be found in smaller amounts in canola and soya bean oils.

SUGAR

According to popular opinion and many food advertising campaigns, glucose and sucrose both help to maintain energy. However, unlike complex carbohydrates, neither glucose nor sucrose in their pure form are essential for a healthy diet, as the body obtains glucose from the gradual breakdown of complex carbohydrate into glucose giving a gradual, continual energy supply.

Excessive intake of refined sugar is one of the most common contributing factors in hypoglycaemia – low blood sugar level (see pages 144–5). Foods high in sugar can cause a rapid rise in blood sugar, which can lead to an excessive production of insulin. People often think that if you have a low blood sugar level you should simply have a cup of tea with a few teaspoons of sugar. However, this could result in more problems. Although there may be a short-term relief in symptoms, it can start a vicious cycle of sugar intake which can lead to excessive insulin production, resulting in low blood sugar and low energy.

The most successful treatment for this type of fatigue is to replace refined carbohydrates with regular complex carbohydrates taken every three to four hours. Complex

AVERAGE NUTRIENTS IN SOME COMMON FOODS

The table below lists a selection of common foods with their approximate nutritional components. You should aim to limit your intake of saturated fats.

Where the fat content figure is followed by an asterisk (*), this indicates that the fat is mostly saturated and therefore the food should be eaten in moderation.

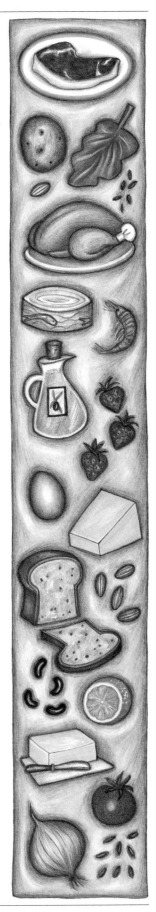

SOURCE	CALORIES	PROTEIN	CARB	FAT	VITAMINS	MINERALS
Liver, calf's, fried 85 g (3 oz)	222 kcal	25.1 g	3.4 g	11.2 g*	A, B_1, B_2, B_3, B_6, B_{12} C, E, M	Cu, Fe, K, P, S, Zn
Sirloin steak, grilled 85 g (3 oz)	176 kcal	27.4 g	0 g	6.0 g*	B_1, B_3, B_6, B_{12}, K	Fe, K, P, S, Zn
Chicken, 85 g (3 oz)	141 kcal	26.9 g	0 g	2.0 g*	B_2, B_3	K, P, S, Zn
Egg, raw, 1 large	82 kcal	6.5 g	0.5 g	4.7 g*	A, B_2, B_{12}, D, E	Fe, P, S, Zn
Salmon, canned 85 g (3 oz)	179 kcal	16.7 g	0 g	7.4 g	A, B_3, B_6, B_{12}, D, E	Ca, F, I, K, P, S, Se, Zn
Prawns, fried 85 g (3 oz)	192 kcal	17.4 g	8.4 g	9.3 g	B_3, B_{12}	Cu, F, Fe, I, K, Mg, Na, P, S, Zn
Olive oil, 1 tbsp	119 kcal	0 g	0 g	12.7 g		
Butter, 1 tbsp	102 kcal	0.1 g	0.1 g	10.4 g*	A	Na
Cheddar cheese, 25 g (1 oz)	113 kcal	7.1 g	0.6 g	8.3 g*	A, B_2, B_{12}, D	Ca, Na, P
Cottage cheese, 85 g (3 oz)	72 kcal	14.4 g	2.4 g	0.3 g	B_2, M	Na, P
Orange, 1 medium	71 kcal	1.1 g	18.1 g	0.3 g	A, B_1, C, M	K
Strawberries, 8 large	55 kcal	1 g	12.5 g	0.7 g	C	Fe, K
Wholewheat bread, 3 slices	168 kcal	7.2 g	33 g	2.1 g	B_1, B_3, B_6, E, K	Mg, Na, P, Zn
Brown rice, cooked 225 g (8 oz)	232 kcal	4.9 g	49.7 g	1.2 g	B_1, B_3, B_6, M	Cu, Fe, K, Mg, Na, P, S, Zn
Almonds, shelled 55 g (2 oz)	340 kcal	10.6 g	11 g	29.2 g	B_1, B_2, B_3, M	Ca, Cu, Fe, K, Mg, P, S, Zn
Kidney beans, cooked 225 g (8 oz)	218 kcal	14.4 g	39.6 g	0.9 g	B_1, M	Cu, Fe, K, Mg, P, Zn
Potatoes, boiled 225 g (8 oz)	163 kcal	4.6 g	36.9 g	0.15 g	B_1, B_3, B_6, C, K	Fe, K, Mg, P
Spinach, blanched 225 g (8 oz)	41 kcal	5.4 g	6.5 g	0.5 g	A, B_1, B_2, C, E, K, M	Ca, Cu, Fe, K, Mg
Tomato, 1 raw	20 kcal	1 g	4.3 g	0.2 g	A, C, K	C
Onion, 225 g (8 oz)	61 kcal	2.5 g	13.7 g	0.2 g	C	K

Key to vitamins B_1 Thiamin, B_2 Riboflavin, B_3 Niacin, B_6 Pyridoxine, M Folic acid
Key to minerals Ca Calcium, Cu Copper, F Fluorine, Fe Iron, I Iodine, K Potassium, Mg Magnesium, Na Sodium, P Phosphorus, S Sulphur, Se Selenium, Zn Zinc

carbohydrates are digested slowly and the resulting glucose is released gradually into the bloodstream, giving a long-lasting supply. This reduces the symptoms of hypoglycaemia, such as fatigue, lethargy and dizziness, with the result that you have more energy throughout the day.

There are some substances in the diet that can have an effect on blood sugar. Caffeine has been shown to increase insulin levels and therefore lower blood sugar. Also, some conditions are made worse by hypoglycaemia, for example PMS (see page 30).

Energy swings

Swings in energy levels that seem to be related to food can be helped by eating regularly – three meals a day with small snacks in between – and basing your diet on complex carbohydrates. Occasionally some nutritional supplements may help in the control of blood sugar, usually in the form of magnesium, chromium and possibly certain B vitamins. These should be prescribed under the guidance of a doctor or dietitian and used in combination with appropriate dietary measures.

SUPPLEMENTS THAT MAY HELP ENERGY

Supplementing the nutrients in your diet with tablets is a practice that has become more popular with increased understanding of our dietary needs. Some doctors and dietitians now prescribe supplements to patients or convalescents if they feel it may help.

Research has concluded that sufferers of illness may benefit from specified supplements, especially if that nutrient was lacking before the onset of illness. However, taking mega-doses of supplements without medical guidance is not advised.

SUPPLEMENT	BENEFITS AND FUNCTIONS	TARGET GROUPS	RDA
Vitamin A	Eyes, skin, growth	Children, smokers	800 µg
Vitamin B complex	Releases energy, promotes healthy skin and nerves, hormone production and antibodies	Pregnant or breastfeeding mothers, those suffering emotional stress	As directed
Vitamin C	Needed for healthy tissues and wound healing, fights infection and is needed to absorb iron	Pregnant or breastfeeding mothers, the elderly, convalescents, drinkers and smokers	60 mg
Folic acid	Helps the production of red blood cells and the reproduction of DNA in foetuses	Women planning pregnancy or who are in early pregnancy	200 µg
Vitamin E	Maintenance of healthy blood, tissue and cells. Helps to reduce damaging effects of pollution	Women taking the contraceptive pill or hormone replacement treatments	10 mg
Iron	Essential for red blood cell development	Menstruating women, vegetarians and vegans	14 mg
Magnesium	Needed for nervous system and muscle movement	Heavy drinkers and those with poor diet	300 mg
Selenium	Protects against skin damage. Helps immune system	The elderly, breastfeeding women, slimmers	None
Zinc	Needed for enzyme production, immune function and normal growth	The elderly and those on a poor or restricted diet	15 mg
Coenzyme Q10	Increases release of energy from food	The elderly, athletes, those on a poor diet	None
Garlic	Good for the heart and immune system	All individuals	None
Gingko biloba	Maintains blood circulation around the body	Those suffering from poor circulation, poor memory and concentration	None
Ginseng	Helps to maintain the natural balance of the body	The elderly, athletes and the busy or stressed	None
GLA (starflower, evening primrose)	Helps the body functions to run smoothly and improves the skin	Premenstrual women with tender breasts	None
Omega 3 (fish oils)	Maintenance of healthy membranes and transport of fats around the body	Those suffering from arthritis, rheumatism or poor circulation	None

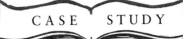
A Constantly Tired Woman

The root of many energy problems lies in a poor diet lacking in vital nutrients, which prevents your body from functioning as well as it should, interrupting the natural course of energy production. With the help of a dietitian, such deficiencies can be corrected through dietary changes and supplements to give you the right balance of energy and nutrients.

Kate is a 32-year-old divorcee with a seven-year-old son. She used to work as a legal secretary, but a year ago she started to get headaches and feel constantly tired and had to work part-time. She put her fatigue down to the strain of dealing with her ex-husband and bringing up her son on her own. Kate was also suffering from PMS, which made her feel weak before her period, prompting chocolate cravings. Her diet consisted of toast for breakfast, a mid-morning sugary snack, sandwiches for lunch, and ready-cooked meals or pies in the evening. She drank 7–8 cups of tea a day. Kate's doctor found nothing wrong physically, but referred her to a PMS clinic where she would be seen by a dietitian.

WHAT SHOULD KATE DO?

When suffering PMS, Kate needs to have regular meals and snacks based on complex carbohydrate to keep the blood sugar up, and prevent the shaky hypoglycaemic-type feelings and headaches. Regular carbohydrate intake should help to banish the chocolate binging. Her whole diet needs to be lower in fat and sugar, and higher in fibre and starch. Research has shown that this is the best diet for PMS. Kate should cut down on caffeinated drinks as this will help to relieve the hypoglycaemic symptoms and encourage restful sleep. She should eat at least five helpings of fruit and vegetables a day, which will provide her with all the important vitamins and minerals she needs.

Action Plan

DIET
Take control of diet and eat for energy. Check the nutritional value of food - select those high in complex carbohydrates and low in sugar and fat.

EATING HABITS
Maintain a constant level of energy by eating regular meals with in-between snacks high in complex carbohydrates. Avoid sugary snacks and stimulants.

EMOTIONAL STRESS
Take control of life. Consider priorities and resolve old disputes that drain so much energy.

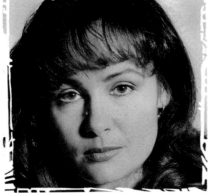

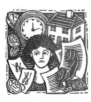

EMOTIONAL STRESS
Letting other people's demands get you down can drain your emotional energy.

DIET
Eating refined and processed foods with little nutritional value can reduce your energy levels in the long run.

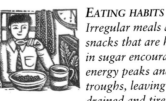

EATING HABITS
Irregular meals and snacks that are high in sugar encourage energy peaks and troughs, leaving you drained and tired.

HOW THINGS TURNED OUT FOR KATE

The PMS clinic recommended a diet of small, regular meals and snacks, based on complex carbohydrates and lots of fruit and vegetables. It was difficult at first – especially cutting down on tea and sweets – but within a couple of weeks Kate had more energy. She now takes her son swimming every week and is looking for a full-time job. She also discussed her marriage problems with a counsellor at the clinic, and now feels more in control.

ENERGY LEVELS THROUGH THE DAY

Regular meals and snacks are vital to give you energy throughout the day. However, the type and quantity of food that you eat can also affect your level of vitality.

Scientists have found that what you eat and drink can affect how tired or alert you are through the day. However, the body plays a big part too, as it has its own natural cycles, known as circadian rhythms. These circadian rhythms go through a constant series of peaks and troughs over 24 hours. There are two big dips in alertness: one at night and a smaller one after lunch at around 2 pm. Certain foods and drinks can exacerbate these troughs. For example, the larger the meal at lunchtime the bigger the post-lunch dip, especially if it is combined with alcohol. Many cultures make use of this natural dip in alertness after lunch by having a siesta.

Some research has concluded that eating a high-protein lunch at midday with a high-carbohydrate low-fat meal in the evening is the best way to maintain alertness. But other studies have failed to support this theory and it remains controversial. Other studies have found a strong relationship between carbohydrate intake, serotonin levels and mood in people on weight-reduction diets. This may help to explain the association between dieting and depression.

Recent work is focusing on a hormone called cholecystokinin which is released by the gut when food is eaten, especially fatty food. Early indications show that this hormone appears to make the research subjects feel more sluggish and inert.

THE IMPORTANCE OF BREAKFAST

Breakfast is a crucial meal because it follows the long overnight fast. Studies have shown that eating breakfast improves cognitive function by affecting short-term metabolic, nervous and hormonal changes. This occurs following the supply of energy and nutrients to the brain. Breakfast has also been found

STAYING ALIVE
The key to all-day energy is to top up your fuel reserves every few hours with carbohydrate snacks. These are slowly absorbed into the system, releasing energy at a steady rate over a long period of time.

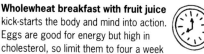

Wholewheat breakfast with fruit juice kick-starts the body and mind into action. Eggs are good for energy but high in cholesterol, so limit them to four a week

Mid-morning fruit and nuts, such as bananas, apples and peanuts, provide a top-up in carbohydrate levels and extra nutrients

Protein-rich lunch, such as meat, fish, beans, cheese or eggs, with fruit or salad fuels you for the afternoon without weighing you down

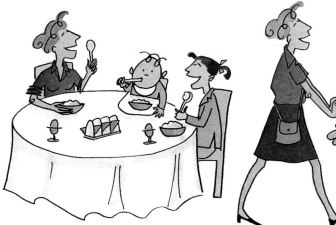

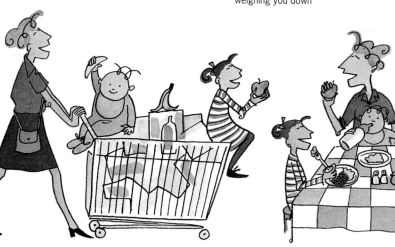

DIET AND NEUROCHEMICALS

Scientists have found links between daily fluctuations in a substance called serotonin and the consumption of carbohydrate-rich foods. Serotonin is a hormone found in tissues, blood and, more importantly, in nerves where it acts as a neurotransmitter – a chemical messenger that improves brain processes, alertness and mood. Research has found that following the ingestion of a meal high in carbohydrate there is an increase in the rate at which the brain produces serotonin. This is thought to be because serotonin is made from the amino acid tryptophan, which is provided in protein foods with other amino acids. Tryptophan needs to compete with all the other amino acids for the same entry points into the brain and is therefore in limited supply. However, foods high in carbohydrates stimulate the release of insulin, which has the effect of clearing away the other amino acids and thus allowing the free passage of tryptophan into the brain. Therefore, carbohydrate-rich diets can help your brain to function properly, enhancing your mood and improving your sleep.

to increase vitamin and mineral intake and improve health. A number of research studies have shown this to be of particular importance in people who are nutritionally at risk, especially children.

If you do not eat breakfast, there will be quite rapid changes in your metabolism; for example, there will be a decline in blood glucose levels that can trigger a stress response which interferes with concentration. If such an effect were to occur regularly it might, for example, undermine a child's progress at school. Several studies have examined the link between brain function and breakfast in schoolchildren; the omission of breakfast seemed particularly to affect the speed and accuracy of information retrieval in the working memory. In Britain and the United States a number of schools have established breakfast programmes to help to alleviate this problem.

DIET FOR SLEEP PROBLEMS

A recent study by Loughborough University found that sleep can be enhanced by eating a light carbohydrate snack just before you go to bed. The carbohydrate increases serotonin production in the brain and also prevents you from feeling hungry during the night. However, you should avoid heavy meals in the evening. Circadian rhythm experts in Liverpool have shown that people who regularly eat late at night are particularly susceptible to digestive disorders and stomach ulcers. The body has trouble entering deep sleep when it is in the first stages of food digestion and the result is fatigue and impaired body functioning.

SOURCES OF COMPLEX CARBOHYDRATES

Complex carbohydrates are found in foods that are rich in wholegrains and starches, such as:

▶ *Wholemeal or granary bread.*

▶ *Rye bread.*

▶ *Wholemeal breakfast cereals, such as bran flakes or porridge oats.*

▶ *Wholemeal pasta.*

▶ *Brown rice.*

▶ *Potatoes.*

▶ *Beans and legumes.*

A glass of milk or fresh fruit or vegetable juice mid afternoon helps to revive your sinking energy levels

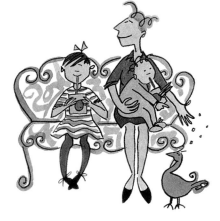

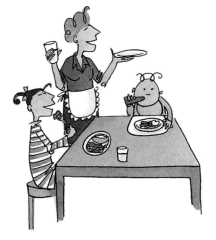

A carbohydrate-rich pasta or potato-based dinner with plenty of lightly cooked vegetables will help to replenish the energy lost during the day

A light carbohydrate snack before bed, such as a few crackers or a slice of wholemeal toast, will help you to sleep soundly

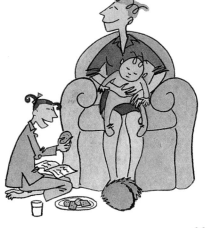

ENERGY LEVELS AND SPECIAL DIETS

If you are following a restricted diet you may face particular challenges in maintaining energy levels. Recognising the problem areas can help you to balance your diet and stay healthy.

Special diets can be adopted for a wide number of reasons, probably the most common being because people simply do not like certain kinds of food. Many give up animal products for moral reasons, and others restrict their diet due to health, for example to avoid an allergen.

VEGETARIANISM

Vegetarian diets have become increasingly popular. A recent survey revealed that over 6 per cent of the British population considered themselves vegetarians – a dramatic 120 per cent increase over the previous five years. There is some concern about the nutritional adequacy of certain plant-based diets but, with planning, most vegetarian diets are consistent with good nutrition and can provide many health benefits.

There are several types of vegetarian diet, of which the most common is lacto-ovo vegetarianism which excludes meat but includes milk, dairy products, and eggs as well as plant foods; lacto vegetarians also exclude eggs. A vegan diet excludes completely all foods that come from animals, including honey. A vegan diet, therefore, is based on cereals and cereal products, pulses, vegetables, fruits, nuts and seeds.

Macronutrients in vegetarian diets

As most plant foods contain more water and fibre and less fat than foods of animal origin, vegetarian diets are usually less dense than conventional diets and for many adults this may help in maintaining an ideal weight. But for growing children, or those with a limited appetite, the bulkiness of vegan and other restrictive vegetarian diets means that there is a risk of not getting enough energy. There have been reports of malnutrition and retarded growth in children fed very restrictive macrobiotic diets. It is important to include plenty of energy-dense foods in the diets of growing children.

There is also concern about whether a vegetarian diet contains enough protein, since plant foods are lower in protein than animal foods. However, the requirement for protein is about 10 per cent of energy intake and many plant foods contain this; for example, pulses average over 25 per cent protein content, and cereals, nuts and seeds over 12 per cent. Surveys have consistently shown that the protein intakes of vegetarians easily meet required levels.

Generally vegetarian diets are low in fat, but recently there has been concern about the balance of the types of fat. Vegan diets can be very high in a particular fatty acid,

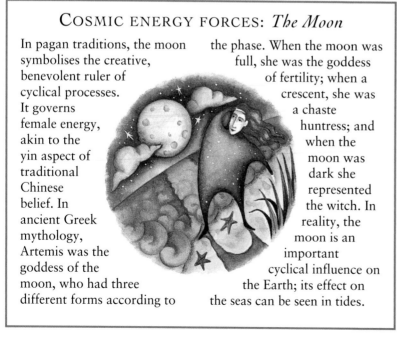

COSMIC ENERGY FORCES: *The Moon*

In pagan traditions, the moon symbolises the creative, benevolent ruler of cyclical processes. It governs female energy, akin to the yin aspect of traditional Chinese belief. In ancient Greek mythology, Artemis was the goddess of the moon, who had three different forms according to the phase. When the moon was full, she was the goddess of fertility; when a crescent, she was a chaste huntress; and when the moon was dark she represented the witch. In reality, the moon is an important cyclical influence on the Earth; its effect on the seas can be seen in tides.

linoleic acid, which is found in sunflower, safflower and corn oil. Too much of this fatty acid can inhibit the body's production of essential fatty acids. The other source of these fatty acids is from oily fish, which vegetarians do not eat. Therefore, it is recommended that vegetarians use soya, rapeseed or olive oil and margarines instead.

Vegetarian diets and vitamins

Studies have shown that vegetarians usually have higher intakes of most vitamins than typical meat eaters. Vegans, however, can be deficient in three vitamins: vitamin D, B_{12} and B_2.

Vitamin D may be a problem because the main sources are either of animal origin – eggs, oily fish, liver – or fortified foods such as margarines and breakfast cereals. The vitamin can be made in skin exposed to sunlight, however, so vegans who spend plenty of time outside should not be deficient.

Vitamin B_{12} is produced by bacteria, fungi and algae and it only accumulates in animals, so a diet based on plants alone tends to be deficient in B_{12}. Recent research has found that many plant-based foods previously thought to have B_{12} do not, so consuming B_{12}-fortified foods is advisable.

HEALTH BENEFITS OF VEGETARIAN DIETS

A vegetarian diet offers many health benefits. Several research studies have shown that they are lower in fat, especially saturated fat, and higher in complex carbohydrate and fibre than conventional diets.

Studies have also shown that vegetarians on average have lower weight and blood fats, and lower rates of heart disease, strokes and certain cancers. Vegetarian and vegan diets have been used successfully to help to lower blood cholesterol, and manage angina, hypertension, obesity, and even asthma and rheumatoid arthritis. Vegetarians may also benefit by avoiding animal-related diseases and food poisoning which have become a problem in recent years.

The major sources of riboflavin (vitamin B_2) are dairy products and meat, and so the dietary intake of this vitamin can be low for vegans, although several studies have shown there to be no major health risks as a result.

ENERGY-RICH FOOD FOR VEGETARIANS

It is crucial that those on vegetarian or vegan diets pay special attention to their energy levels. The following foods contain much of the goodness that vegetarians need.

▶ *Nuts and nut spreads.*

▶ *Pulses and dried fruits.*

▶ *Tofu, soya milk and other soya products.*

▶ *Vegetable oils.*

▶ *For the lacto-ovo vegetarian: eggs, milk and dairy products.*

MINERALS AND THE VEGETARIAN DIET

Minerals can be limited in vegetarian diets, mostly because they are not always available in plant products. Mineral intake can also be affected by phytates, found in wholegrains, which can bind with minerals, such as iron. When cereals are refined phytate is removed, and with it some of the minerals, so to maintain good levels of mineral intake try to eat wholegrain products.

HEALTHY CHOICES
The protein foods shown here provide 100 mg calcium – more than the RDA – as well as 1 mg iron and 1 mg zinc. They are all inexpensive and suitable for both vegetarian and vegan diets.

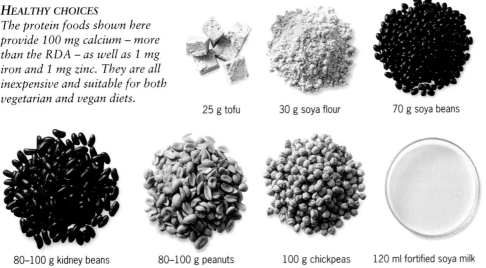

25 g tofu   30 g soya flour   70 g soya beans

80–100 g kidney beans   80–100 g peanuts   100 g chickpeas   120 ml fortified soya milk

DIETARY NEEDS FOR THE UNDERWEIGHT

If you are recovering from illness or have been chronically underweight you should eat as healthily as possible while consistently gaining weight. A dietitian can help you to target your weight gain per week, although you should not attempt to regain weight too fast as this could cause metabolism imbalances and lead to other health problems. Gently add calorie-rich foods to your basic diet.

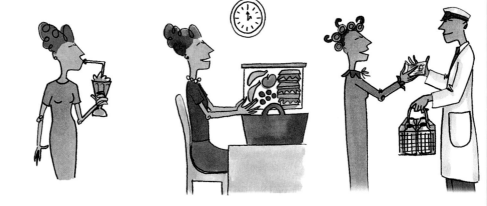

Eat plenty of high calorie and nutritious snacks including bananas, avocados, nuts, dried fruits and fruit smoothies

Eat regularly and never miss a meal. This will keep your energy levels topped up and build up your nutrient levels and energy stores

Have plenty of dairy products which are high in protein and nutrients and also in fat, such as a glass of milk or a milk shake

DIABETES

Diabetes mellitus is caused by a shortage of insulin (see page 142). There are two types of diabetes: insulin-dependent diabetes (IDD) which is treated by injection of insulin, and non-insulin-dependent diabetes (NIDD), which is treated through diet and drugs. Generally speaking, it is younger diabetics who need to inject insulin (IDD), while older sufferers have some insulin but their bodies fail to respond to it sufficiently so they need to control their diet (NIDD).

The aim of dietary treatment is to stop the harmful symptoms of diabetes by keeping blood glucose levels as close to normal as possible. It is also important to reduce the risk of hypoglycaemia in IDD. Dietary measures are fully covered on page 143.

In dietary terms, the energy content of the diet, when related to the individual's requirements, has probably the greatest effect on long-term diabetic control. It has been estimated that around 75 per cent of NIDD sufferers are overweight, and research has shown that reducing energy and therefore calorie intake in the overweight diabetic is effective in helping the blood glucose return to normal.

A high complex or unrefined-carbohydrate diet has been recommended for people with diabetes since 1982. The British Diabetic Association suggests that carbohydrate should provide between 50 and 55 per cent of energy. The fibre content seems to be essential, and the British Diabetic Association recommends that a total of 30 grams of dietary fibre should be eaten daily.

CHROMIUM DEFICIENCY AND DIABETES

Chromium regulates the action and efficiency of insulin in the body. A number of studies conducted in the United States in the 1990s found that the body's chromium status decreases with age, especially in men. This suggests that some of the diseases associated with ageing, such as non-insulin-dependent diabetes and heart disease, may be linked to the age-related decrease in chromium levels. Chromium is found in wholegrain cereals and, therefore, a diet high in refined carbohydrate could result in chromium deficiency. Chromium supplements have been shown to improve diabetics' insulin control.

ENERGY BOOST

Broccoli is one of the most nutrient-rich vegetables and is surprisingly high in protein. Other nutrients include vitamin C, B_2 and folic acid.

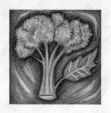

Losing Weight

A weight-loss plan can be a tremendous strain if you are a food lover. However, many people also suffer from a more fundamental loss of energy with a decrease in calorie intake. This can be remedied by a high-carbohydrate, low-fat diet plan.

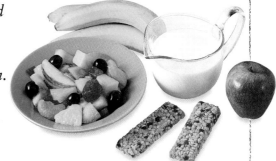

The key to any diet is to reduce the intake of fuel so that you use up the reserves that you have stored as fat in your body. The best way to do this, without compromising your health and energy levels, is by adopting a high-nutrient, low-fat, low-sugar diet, keeping you satisfied and healthy without so many calories. Low-calorie alternatives to

many foods are now widely available, allowing you to eat the same foods with lower energy values. However, to keep your energy levels high, you need to add plenty of fibre and complex carbohydrate to your diet, helping you to get through the day without your blood sugar levels falling too low and your stomach rumbling.

KEEPING YOUR ENERGY LEVELS HIGH
Eating snacks throughout the day will help to keep the hunger pains at bay and your energy levels high. However, you must make sure that your food choices are low in fat and high in nutrients and complex carbohydrates.

CHOOSING LOW-FAT, LOW-SUGAR, HIGH-CARBOHYDRATE ALTERNATIVES

Complex carbohydrates are absorbed slowly by your digestive system, maintaining a stream of nutrients and energy pouring into your system over a long period of time, and preventing you from feeling hungry or

lacking in energy. These should be chosen above sugary or fatty foods which may give you instant energy boosts but will tire you out in the long term. Healthier alternatives to many foods are described below.

SUBSTITUTE	INSTEAD OF	WHY MAKE THE CHANGE?
Skimmed and semi-skimmed milk	Full-fat milk	Milk is an important constituent of a normal diet, although it is extremely fattening, and milk fat is saturated and bad for the heart and arteries
Low-sugar cereal bars	Chocolate bars	Cereals provide complex carbohydrates to release energy gradually
Low-sugar soft drinks	Soft drinks	Sugar in soft drinks unbalances your blood sugar levels in the long run
Low-calorie dessert	Cakes, trifles, etc	Helps weight loss and health while still satisfying a sweet tooth
Trimmed or extra lean meat	Fatty meat	The fat in meat is saturated – fattening and bad for your health
Bran cereal	Cornflakes	Increasing the fibre in your diet fills you up and provides the nutrients that you need without adding extra calories
Steamed or grilled foods	Fried foods	Frying food increases nutrient loss and adds needless calories
Reduced-sugar jams and biscuits	Jams and biscuits	Reducing sugar helps to balance your blood sugar and energy levels
Fruit salad	Cake	Fruit provides plenty of nutrients and fibre without the calories
Salads and vegetables	Potato crisps and chips	Vegetables can fill you up with fewer calories and more nutrients
Low-calorie sauces and salad dressings	Sauces and salad dressings	Sauces are often misleadingly high in calories and fat
A piece of fruit or dried fruit	Potato crisps	Potato crisps are low in carbohydrate and very high in fat

THE ENERGY NUTRIENTS

Intakes of various nutrients will vary from person to person depending on many factors, including height and weight, age, metabolism, illnesses, physical condition and lifestyle.

The human body needs a whole range of vitamins, minerals and other nutrients to keep it operating efficiently and healthily. But some of these nutrients are of more importance to metabolism and energy production than others, and these energy nutrients are described in the pages that follow. Understanding how each nutrient works within the system and the effects of deficiency on your energy levels can help you to ensure that any energy problems you may be experiencing are not being caused by nutrient deficiency.

Some of the best food sources for each nutrient are shown, as well as a brief description of the main food groups in which the nutrient can be found. The food sources, as well as the recommended dietary requirements where appropriate, are given in either mg (milligrams, one-thousandth of a gram) or µg (micrograms, one millionth of a gram) depending upon the quantity denomination. A recipe suggestion shows you how to increase the nutrient in your diet in an easy and delicious way. After all, eating healthily does not mean depriving yourself of flavour and the enjoyment of food.

A large and growing body of research is currently being amassed which shows the links between nutrient deficiencies and a lack of energy. Magnesium supplements, for example, have been found to significantly alleviate fatigue problems in those who are slightly deficient in this mineral. The B vitamins have been widely recognised by medical experts for their beneficial contribution to metabolism and psychological health, which in turn raises energy levels. Advances in our understanding of neurotransmitters have led medical researchers to harness amino acids, such as carnitine, for their energy-boosting qualities. Coenzyme Q10 has generated great interest since it was discovered to improve metabolism substantially. New and exciting links between energy and micronutrients are emerging in research centres throughout the world, and more are expected in the future.

THE STRUCTURE OF VITAMINS

All of the vitamins have complex molecular structures which consist mainly of the elements carbon, oxygen, nitrogen and hydrogen. Their structure allows them to form bonds with other molecules within food. On cooking many of the bonds weaken, allowing the vitamins to drain out.

FAT-SOLUBLE VITAMINS
Vitamins A, D, E and K are fat-soluble – they are absorbed into the lymph and any excess is stored in fatty tissues.

WATER-SOLUBLE VITAMINS
Vitamins B and C are absorbed directly into the blood and any excess is excreted with urine.

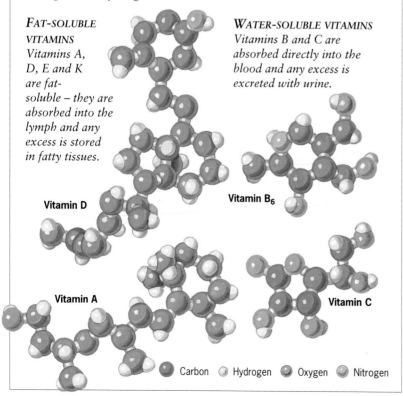

Vitamin D

Vitamin B₆

Vitamin A

Vitamin C

Carbon Hydrogen Oxygen Nitrogen

HOW YOUR BODY USES VITAMINS AND MINERALS

Although most vitamins and minerals are required throughout the body for general functioning, many play a specific role – or number of roles – enabling different systems to function properly. However, the knock-on effect of one part functioning poorly as a result of nutrient deficiency has a chance of affecting the entire body. The interaction between minerals and vitamins is complex and a deficiency or excess in one is likely to lead to many other problems. All of the following vitamins and minerals need to be obtained through the diet with the exception of vitamin D, which can be absorbed from sunlight through the skin, and vitamin K, which is partially produced by bacteria in the gut.

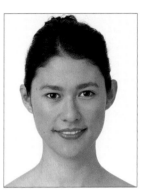

Skin and hair need vitamins A, B_2, B_3, B_6 and B_{12}, biotin, sulphur and zinc. Healthy eyes and eyesight benefit from vitamin A and zinc. Healthy teeth need vitamins C and D, calcium, phosphorus, fluorine and magnesium

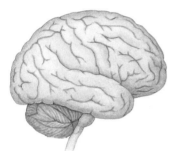

Nervous system functioning can be strengthened by the following nutrients: vitamins B_1, B_6, B_{12} and E, biotin, calcium, potassium, sodium and magnesium

Cardiovascular strength is a crucial constituent of good health. Important nutrients include vitamin B_1, calcium, copper, magnesium, sodium, potassium and selenium

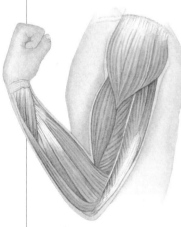

Energy production can be improved by: vitamins B_1, B_2, B_3, B_5, biotin, calcium, chromium, copper, iodine, iron, magnesium, phosphorus and potassium. Proper muscle functioning depends on vitamin B_1, calcium, magnesium, potassium and sodium

*VITAL BALANCE
The correct balance of minerals and vitamins is needed to ensure proper body functioning. A healthy and balanced diet should provide you with your daily needs.*

Healthy bones need vitamins A, C and D, calcium, copper, fluorine, phosphorus and magnesium. Babies and children need more of these nutrients for healthy growth

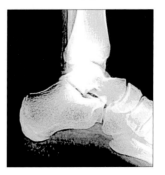

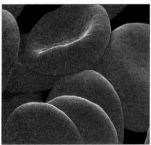

Healthy blood cell formation is assisted by vitamins B_6, B_{12}, E, folic acid, copper and iron. Blood clotting depends on vitamin K and calcium

▼▼

Thiamin

Thiamin, also known as vitamin B_1, plays a crucial role in converting carbohydrates and fats into energy, and in preventing the build-up of toxins which are natural by-products of metabolism in the body.

THE DISCOVERY OF THIAMIN

Beri-beri was first mentioned by a Dutch naval doctor in 1873 who found that the incidence of the disease decreased by reducing white rice in the diet. In the 1890s, Christiaan Eijkman, a physician in the Dutch East Indies, found that beri-beri symptoms could be cured by adding the polishings of rice (the part removed in processing) to the diet. In 1911, biochemist Casimir Funk, working at the Lister Institute in London, isolated what he termed a 'vitamine' which prevented beri-beri. However, what he had actually discovered was niacin. Two Dutch scientists working in Java, Jansen and Donath, eventually identified thiamin in 1926.

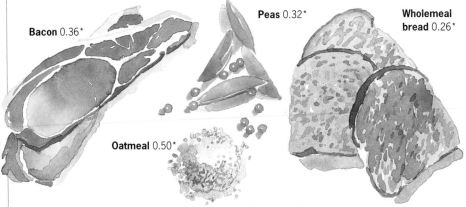

Bacon 0.36*

Peas 0.32*

Wholemeal bread 0.26*

Oatmeal 0.50*

*mg per 100 g

The amount of thiamin the body needs is related to the amount and type of energy foods consumed, particularly carbohydrate. High-carbohydrate diets require more thiamin to metabolise than high-fat diets. There are also a number of naturally occurring substances with antithiamin activity, such as tea, coffee and a number of fruits and vegetables including blackberries, blackcurrants, beetroot, spinach and cabbage. Antithiamin substances are also present in raw fish and shellfish, but are destroyed by cooking.

In less developed countries thiamin deficiency – known as beri-beri, which is Singhalese for extreme weakness – is usually due to diets of white rice and/or eating raw fish. In developed countries alcoholism is the main cause of deficiency, and usually there is a deficiency of several nutrients, not just thiamin.

Thiamin is crucial to the body's energy-production system. Deficiency leads to rapid deterioration in both heart and skeletal muscle function, problems

SOURCES AND REQUIREMENTS

Sources
Thiamin is found in foods of both vegetable and animal origin. Particularly good sources include wholegrains, pork, beef, peas, beans, lentils, soya products, marmite and brown rice. Refined foods, such as white rice and white flour, have substantially reduced levels.

Dietary requirements
The requirement for thiamin depends on calorie intake, but ranges from 1 to 1.8 mg per day for adults.

with brain and nerve function, loss of appetite and weight loss, and associated fatigue symptoms. Thiamin deficiency may be a contributing factor in many non-specific conditions such as anorexia, weight loss, fatigue and depression.

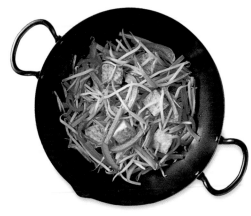

TOFU WITH CHINESE VEGETABLES
Slice a spring onion, a green pepper and a carrot and stir fry in a hot pan for a few minutes. Add diced tofu and fry for a further 5 minutes. Add a few handfuls of beansprouts, splash in some soy sauce and cook briefly until the beansprouts become slightly soft. Tofu and other soya products are rich in thiamin.

▲▲

Riboflavin

Riboflavin, also known as vitamin B_2, was discovered in the 1930s when it was isolated from yeast extract. It is essential to the healthy functioning of the liver and the production of energy by the body.

Riboflavin plays a major role in the formation of a number of enzymes that are mainly found in the liver. These enzymes help with the removal of hydrogen molecules and the introduction of oxygen molecules. During this process certain essential substances are metabolised and energy is released.

Riboflavin is crucial in the metabolism of carbohydrates, proteins and fats, as well as in the oxidation of many other substances. It also enhances the metabolism of vitamin B_6. This is why some people with riboflavin deficiency have vitamin B_6 deficiency symptoms and signs.

Riboflavin deficiency is not life threatening as the body is efficient at re-utilising the vitamin. Riboflavin is released as a by-product of its own metabolism, and only a very small amount is excreted.

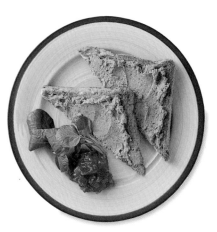

CHICKEN LIVER PATE WITH WHOLEMEAL TOAST
This can be eaten as a nutritious snack between meals, as an appetiser or as a meal in itself. The pâté can be bought ready-made, or you may prefer to make your own. Liver is one of the best sources of riboflavin and other nutrients.

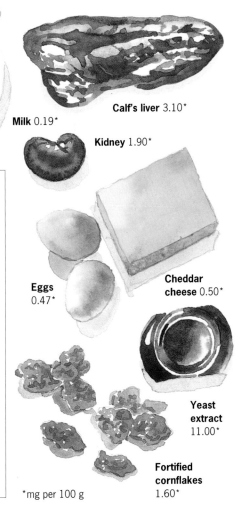

Milk 0.19*

Calf's liver 3.10*

Kidney 1.90*

Eggs 0.47*

Cheddar cheese 0.50*

Yeast extract 11.00*

Fortified cornflakes 1.60*

*mg per 100 g

SYMPTOMS OF DEFICIENCY

Early symptoms include sore and burning lips and tongue. These can also occur in vitamin B_6 deficiency, but dryness, cracking and peeling of the lips is a particular characteristic of lack of riboflavin. The skin on the face becomes red, greasy and scaly, especially at the sides of the nose. Also, unlike vitamin B_6 shortage, there may be a sensitivity to light and other eye irritations. People with riboflavin deficiency complain of burning feet.

SOURCES AND REQUIREMENTS

Sources
Major food sources of riboflavin include yeast extract, dairy produce, cereals, meats (especially offal) and some green leafy vegetables. Approximately one-third of the average intake in the UK is from one source – milk. Riboflavin is fairly stable with heat but deteriorates on exposure to light.

Dietary requirements
Requirements vary considerably depending on the person's stage of growth. Infants require about 0.6 mg per day and this increases up to 1.8 mg for teenagers. Adults require 1.2 mg per day, and up to 1.6 mg per day is needed for pregnant women, and 2.0 mg per day for breastfeeding women.

Niacin

Niacin, also known as vitamin B₃ or nicotinic acid, plays an important part in the formation of certain enzymes which are involved in glucose and carbohydrate metabolism and energy production.

PELLAGRA EPIDEMICS

The first research into niacin was conducted in the 18th century when pellagra was a common disease in Italy and Spain (the name *pellagra* is Italian for 'skin that is rough'). It was found that adding milk or eggs to the diet could alleviate symptoms quickly.

Widespread evidence of niacin deficiency emerged throughout the southern United States during the late 19th and early 20th centuries. This was believed to result from a diet based on maize (corn) and other cereals. Nicotinic acid is actually present in maize, but in a form that is not available for human absorption. Interestingly, the Mexican method of preparing corn for tortillas causes chemical changes which allow the niacin to become available.

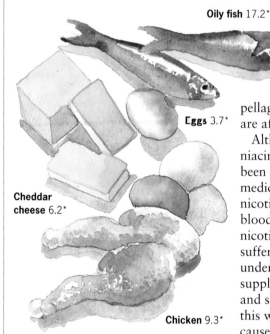

Oily fish 17.2*

Eggs 3.7*

Cheddar cheese 6.2*

Chicken 9.3*

*mg niacin equivalent per 100 g

pellagra about twice as many women are affected than men.

Although most people have enough niacin in their diet, supplements have been found to help a number of medical conditions. Niacin in its nicotinic form can help to lower blood cholesterol levels, and in its nicotinamide form can help arthritis sufferers. Research has been undertaken into the use of niacin supplements in psychotic treatments, and schizophrenics may be helped in this way. However, high doses can cause liver disorders, peptic ulcers and glucose intolerance.

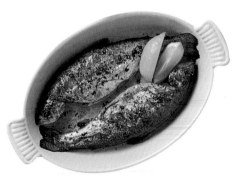

BAKED TROUT WITH LEMON
Blend lemon juice with olive oil and garlic. Spoon the mixture over the fish and place in a medium oven for 20 minutes, turning halfway through the cooking. Serve with lemon wedges and a crisp, green salad. Oily fish, such as trout, tuna and sardines, are all excellent sources of niacin.

There are two main forms of vitamin B₃: niacin, also known as nicotinic acid, is very closely related to the other compound, nicotinamide. Classic deficiency produces a condition known as pellagra with the three major symptoms of dermatitis, diarrhoea and dementia – commonly referred to as the three Ds. Niacin can be synthesised from the amino acid tryptophan (see page 107). Research has found that 60 mg of tryptophan provides 1 mg of niacin. Many foods are therefore described in terms of their 'niacin equivalent', which is dependent on the content of both niacin and tryptophan.

The synthesis of tryptophan into niacin is reduced by oestrogen, which explains why in epidemics of

SOURCES AND REQUIREMENTS

Sources
Major food sources include fish (especially oily fish), meat (particularly beef and offal), milk, fish and wholegrains. Populations that rely heavily on maize are at risk of niacin deficiency because the niacin in maize is in a form that cannot be absorbed by the human digestive system.

Dietary requirements
An average intake of about 15 mg a day for women and 19 mg a day for men should be sufficient.

Pantothenic acid

Pantothenic acid, or vitamin B_5, is one of the lesser-known vitamins. Like the other B vitamins, it plays a major role in energy production and is required for the metabolism of carbohydrates, fats and amino acids.

Pantothenic acid has been found to be particularly important for the proper functioning of the adrenal hormones, and is often connected with a reduction in stress due to better adrenal functioning.

Experimental studies producing a deficiency of pantothenic acid have found that signs of deficiency take several weeks to appear. Studies of intake and excretion suggest that the body has considerable stores which can be drawn upon in times of a dietary deficiency. The symptoms of deficiency include fatigue, headaches, weakness, impaired muscle coordination and muscle cramps.

The only known non-experimental cases were prisoners of war in the Far East during the Second World War, who had a condition known as 'burning-foot syndrome'. Although not tested, it is assumed that this was a result of vitamin B_5 deficiency.

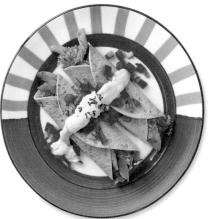

SPICY CHICKEN TORTILLAS
Quick-fry strips of chicken breast in a little olive oil, adding the juice of a lime at the end. Place in a tortilla filled with fresh shredded lettuce. Add salsa and soured cream to taste. All ingredients provide pantothenic acid.

*mg per 100 g

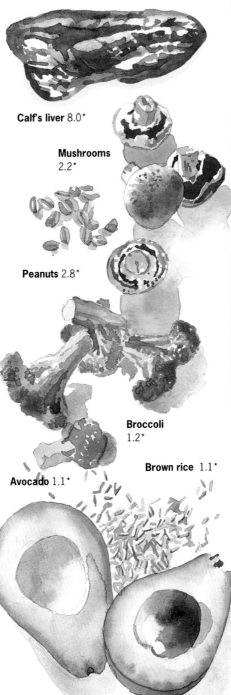

Calf's liver 8.0*

Mushrooms 2.2*

Peanuts 2.8*

Broccoli 1.2*

Brown rice 1.1*

Avocado 1.1*

SOURCES AND REQUIREMENTS

Sources
Pantothenic acid is widely distributed. Its name originates from the Greek *pantos*, which means 'everywhere'. Particularly high levels are found in eggs, liver and mushrooms.

Dietary requirements
There is no official RDA since deficiency is rare. However, 4–7 mg per day is considered adequate for the average adult.

B VITAMINS

The B group of vitamins is a collection of essential nutrients that have certain characteristics in common. Most are water soluble and are essential to the series of steps in the body's metabolism that leads to the release of energy from carbohydrates and fats in the diet or from body stores.

Although severe deficiencies are relatively rare, there is substantial evidence that mild or moderate deficiencies do occur and are related to fatigue.

Those considered more at risk of fatigue or psychological problems associated with B vitamin shortages include alcoholics, the elderly, those eating a poor or restricted diet, and those suffering depression or other mental disorders.

Vitamin B_6

Also known as pyridoxine, vitamin B_6 is a major player in the metabolism of amino acids and is necessary for the formation of haemoglobin in the blood, crucial for maintaining energy levels.

THE B VITAMINS AND PSYCHIATRIC PROBLEMS

Many studies have examined vitamin B deficiencies in groups of people with psychiatric problems. Dr Carney of Northwick Park Hospital, London, showed that patients diagnosed with anxiety, depression or schizophrenia had a 50 per cent chance of being deficient in one or more B vitamins. He linked depression with vitamin B_2 and B_6 deficiencies and some doctors recommend vitamin B supplements for those suffering from mental illnesses.

B vitamins have also become a relatively popular alternative treatment for premenstrual syndrome and the symptoms of menopause.

Vitamin B_6 is important to many different functions, primarily for its role in amino acid reactions that are crucial to metabolic processes. Deficiency is rarely bad enough to produce definite symptoms, although minor and temporary symptoms may occur, including loss of energy and inability to concentrate. Deficiency may adversely affect the metabolism of tryptophan and methionine, thus influencing the biochemical status and contributing to depression and other psychological imbalances.

The only known incidence of deficiency occurred in the UK during the 1950s, when some babies were fed on a milk preparation that had been overheated during manufacture. The symptoms included severe convulsions, believed to be caused by the impairment of a regulatory neurotransmitter.

Taking a vitamin B_6 supplement is thought by some to improve mood. In a recent study, a group of 129 young healthy adults took various vitamin supplements for a year and

SOURCES AND REQUIREMENTS

Sources
Vitamin B_6 is found widely in food, particularly in meat, fish, eggs and wholegrains.

Dietary requirements
There are no official recommended requirements since deficiency is rare. Deficiencies are more often due to a lack of riboflavin, with similar symptoms.

some reported better mental health, more composure and significantly improved mood. The benefits were associated with improved vitamin B_2 and vitamin B_6 status. However, further research has yet to establish any firm link.

To date, no substantiated research suggests that overdosing on vitamin B_6 can cause any detrimental side effects.

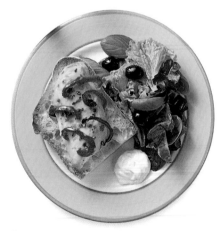

GRILLED CHICKEN AND PEPPER ROSETTI
Marinate skinned chicken breast in lemon juice, garlic and olive oil for a few hours, then place under a hot grill with slices of pepper until cooked. Serve on toasted Italian bread with mixed salad leaves, basil, olives and a smidgen of mayonnaise. Chicken, as well as other meats, is a good source of vitamin B_6.

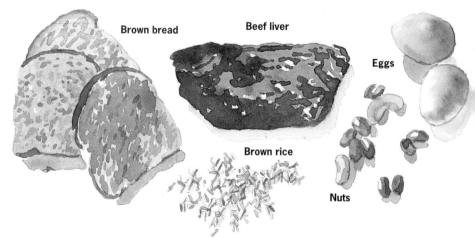

Brown bread

Beef liver

Eggs

Brown rice

Nuts

Vitamin B$_{12}$

Vitamin B$_{12}$, sometimes called cyanocabalamin, is found only in animal-based foods. It is essential to humans for the production of energy and a variety of other functions, including red blood cell production.

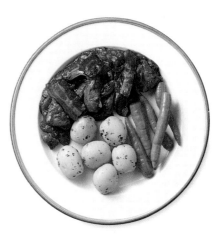

Vitamin B$_{12}$ in the diet is absorbed by the small intestine, but it requires the presence of a compound known as intrinsic factor, which is produced by the stomach. This combines chemically with vitamin B$_{12}$, enabling it to be absorbed in the lower part of the small intestine. Vitamin B$_{12}$ is then transported to the liver where it is stored. It works closely with folic acid to produce red blood cells.

Conditions affecting the stomach and the lower part of the small intestine can cause a vitamin B$_{12}$ deficiency. However, as the body's stores of vitamin B$_{12}$ can last for three to six years, a clinically obvious deficiency takes some time.

Vitamin B$_{12}$ deficiency can be inherited through a rare genetic defect, known as pernicious anaemia. It is caused by a lack of intrinsic factor and is characterised by large, immature red blood cells and damage to the nervous system. It tends to be associated with blue eyes and premature greying of the hair.

CALF'S LIVER AND BACON
Fry strips of bacon with a sliced onion. When nearly cooked, add strips of liver and fry for two minutes. Make a gravy by adding a tablespoonful of plain flour to the juices, stir in and then add stock.

SOURCES AND REQUIREMENTS

Sources

The best sources of vitamin B$_{12}$ are liver, meat and shellfish. Other sources include fish, dairy produce, eggs and yeast. Vitamin B$_{12}$ does not occur in vegetable foods, and therefore those on a strictly vegan diet should consider taking a supplement.

Dietary requirements

The requirements for vitamin B$_{12}$ are minimal, particularly as the body conserves most of the vitamin. For pregnant women, at least 1 microgram (µg) per day is recommended.

Vitamin B$_{12}$ has been traditionally prescribed for fatigue disorders, although a clear link has not been made unless there is a marked deficiency that needs to be supplemented.

*µg per 100 g

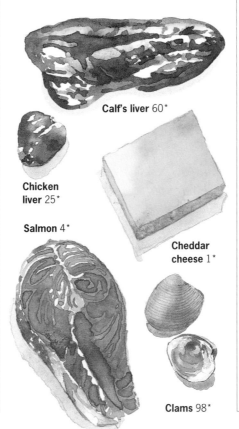

Calf's liver 60*

Chicken liver 25*

Salmon 4*

Cheddar cheese 1*

Clams 98*

SYMPTOMS OF DEFICIENCY

A shortage of vitamin B$_{12}$ results in an anaemia similar to that produced by a deficiency of folic acid (see page 102), with symptoms such as exhaustion, shortness of breath on exertion and pale skin. There are also characteristic changes in the nervous system, including numbness and tingling in the hands and feet, clumsiness and difficulty walking. Although difficult to diagnose, early treatment is vital to prevent serious and potentially permanent damage to the nervous system.

Mild symptoms may also be experienced by vegetarians and vegans. Some vegan products are labelled high in vitamin B$_{12}$ but, although the product may well contain the vitamin, it is not always in a form that can be absorbed by the human gut.

Folic acid

The metabolism of folic acid and vitamin B_{12} are closely linked. Folic acid is vital for the functioning of the central nervous system and DNA replication, making it essential for healthy foetal development.

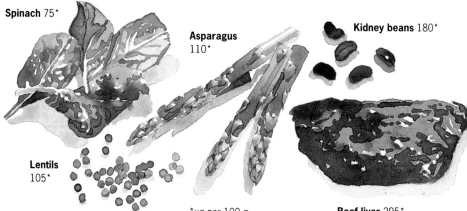

Spinach 75*

Asparagus 110*

Kidney beans 180*

Lentils 105*

*μg per 100 g

Beef liver 295*

FOLIC ACID AND PREGNANCY

Folic acid has been found to be particularly important before and during pregnancy. This is because of its role in cell division and DNA synthesis – without folic acid cells do not divide properly and foetal development may be impaired. This can lead to a number of birth defects, including neural tube defects such as spina bifida. Pregnant women are therefore recommended to take supplements to ensure there is no deficiency. There is no evidence to suggest that taking more folic acid than needed improves foetal development. Prematurely born infants are also given folic acid supplements to ensure a stable and healthy growth.

TUSCAN BEAN SOUP
Chop and lightly fry some broccoli, onion and garlic in a saucepan. Add a tin of tomatoes and some cooked mixed beans, boiling water, mixed herbs and a splash of red wine. Season and simmer for 20 minutes. Broccoli, beans and other legumes are rich in folic acid.

Folic acid is absorbed from the diet and transported to the liver where it is metabolised and stored. Mild deficiency of folic acid may be fairly common in the general population and the symptoms can include anorexia, insomnia and irritability, and recurrent mouth ulcers. Only the more severe folic acid deficiencies show up as anaemia. A shortage of either vitamin B_{12} or folic acid will eventually result in anaemia which produces tiredness, shortness of breath and pale skin as well as depression and, in extreme cases, nerve damage. Cracking of the corners of the mouth has been linked with folic acid deficiency, but this is also a sign of vitamin B_2, B_6 and iron deficiency.

The main groups at risk of deficiency are pregnant or breastfeeding women and young infants. This is because of the folic acid needed for DNA replication and growth. Since nitrates may destroy folic acid under acid conditions, there is a fear that nitrate-polluted water may also lead to deficiency.

SOURCES AND REQUIREMENTS

Sources
The best sources include liver, wholegrain cereals and green vegetables – the name folic comes from the word foliage. Folic acid can be easily destroyed by cooking, but cooking with foods high in vitamin C can prevent this.

Dietary requirements
The RDA for folic acid is 200 micrograms (μg) per day for men and 180 for women. Women who are planning a pregnancy should take 400 micrograms every day, and should continue until they are into their 12th week of pregnancy.

Folic acid antagonists, such as methotrexate, are used in chemotherapy to prevent the folic acid from synthesising cancer cells, and thus slowing its spread. This may also cause deficiency symptoms.

Choline

Choline is essential in human nutrition. Its action is related to that of the B vitamins as it is crucial in the production of energy from carbohydrates. It also acts as a neurotransmitter which can improve mood.

Choline is a constituent of lecithin, a fat emulsifier necessary for the proper metabolism of fats. Without choline, fats become trapped in the liver and can block proper metabolism, which can lead to major disorders in the liver and kidneys and cause massive energy loss.

It also acts as a neurotransmitter in the brain. Low levels have been linked to bad memory, poor concentration and Alzheimer's.

Deficiency symptoms are rarely seen in humans, although in many animals a choline deficiency leads to serious liver and kidney disorders.

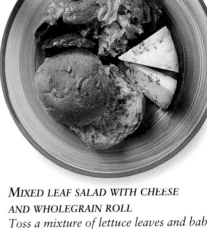

MIXED LEAF SALAD WITH CHEESE AND WHOLEGRAIN ROLL
Toss a mixture of lettuce leaves and baby spinach leaves with French dressing and serve with a wedge of your favourite cheese and a wholegrain roll. All of the ingredients provide choline.

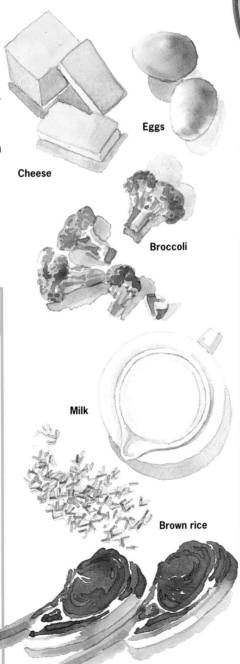

Eggs

Cheese

Broccoli

Milk

Brown rice

Lamb chops

SOURCES AND REQUIREMENTS

Sources
Choline is abundant in a range of foods, particularly eggs, meat and dairy products, but also wholegrain cereals and green vegetables. In diets containing protein, choline can also be made in the human body.

Unfortunately, rich sources of choline tend also to be high in cholesterol, which should be avoided. Dietitians advise that a low level of cholesterol is allowable – such as 300 mg of cholesterol each day, the equivalent of four eggs a week – although not in all cases.

Dietary requirements
There are no recommended daily allowances since deficiency is rare.

THE MOOD-ALTERING INDUSTRY

There is a growing interest in the food and drink industry to develop products claiming psychoactive effects. Choline is thought to have the potential, when channelled properly, to change mood due to its effect of raising neurotransmitter levels, believed to encourage feelings of contentment and relaxation. A company in the United States, Life Force Trading, have advertised a range of soft drinks that 'allow you to take control of your neurochemistry', which includes the 'Gourmet Choline Cooler'. It cannot be assumed, however, that the inclusion of a neurotransmitter precursor in a food or drink will necessarily endow the product with mood-altering properties.

Vitamin C

Studies carried out in the last ten years have shown a strong relationship between vitamin C intake and fatigue. Deficiency can cause a loss of energy and dull aching muscular pains in the legs.

SCURVY AND VITAMIN C DEFICIENCY

The earliest sign that a deficiency of micronutrients could cause a lack of energy came in 1753 from Dr James Lind, a British naval surgeon who was working with cases of scurvy in sailors. Lind observed that the first symptom was a 'listlessness to action or an aversion to any sort of exercise … much fatigue … breathlessness and panting'. He also noted that sailors under stress developed scurvy faster than those who were not under stress, despite having similar diets. It is now well known that stress increases the body's requirements for many micronutrients. Although vitamin C had not been isolated at the time, citrus fruits were known to prevent scurvy and were therefore regularly issued to sailors.

Vitamin C has many roles in the body. It is required for maintaining strength in blood vessels, the metabolism of cholesterol, detoxification of drugs, and maintaining the immune system. Vitamin C has an effect on energy because it is involved in the production of a substance called carnitine (see opposite).

Vitamin C in vegetables is easily destroyed by cooking, and people living in institutions, including old people's homes, are at risk of deficiency due to the overcooking of vegetables and insufficient fresh fruit. In Western society intakes of vitamin C are generally good. In Britain, the average daily intake for adults is 60–70 mg and as little as 5 mg will prevent scurvy, but early mild deficiency can occur more easily, and may cause depression, lethargy, hypochondriasis and hysteria prior to more serious symptoms. Aches and pains, particularly in the legs, are a

common feature of mild deficiency. People who drink a lot of alcohol or smoke may break down vitamin C more quickly and need more. Vitamin C requirement can be raised by stress, acute illness, infections, or where there is an increased need for tissue repair or healing, such as after an operation or burn.

SOURCES AND REQUIREMENTS

Sources
The highest contributions to vitamin C intake in the UK are from fresh fruit and fruit juices, but potatoes are also an important source because large quantities are traditionally eaten.

Dietary requirements
A minimum of 40 mg per day is recommended, but you should have more if you drink alcohol or smoke.

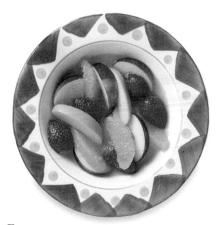

FRUIT SALAD
Mix six halved strawberries with an apple and an orange, cut into bite-sized pieces. Add fruit juice and clear honey to taste. Strawberries are one of the best sources of vitamin C; apples and oranges are also both rich in this nutrient.

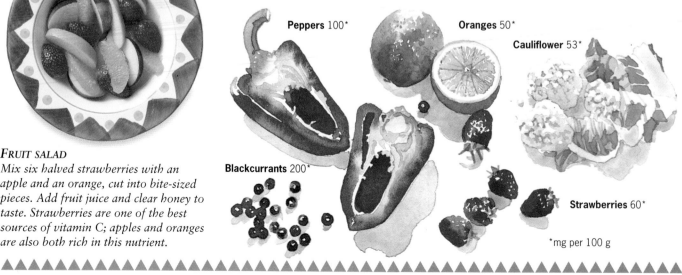

Peppers 100*

Oranges 50*

Cauliflower 53*

Blackcurrants 200*

Strawberries 60*

*mg per 100 g

Carnitine

Carnitine is an amino acid which plays an important role in energy production, enabling the muscle cells to convert fat into energy. When carnitine levels are low, there will be a reduction in muscle function.

Carnitine is an amino acid which enables fatty acids in the body to cross into the inner membrane of mitochondria (tiny energy factories within each cell), so they can be transformed into energy. The more and better quality carnitine is in the system, the more efficiently fat will be turned into energy.

Carnitine synthesis needs adequate vitamin C and iron, and those with a poor diet or a high alcohol intake may suffer from a deficiency of either of these, leading to poor carnitine synthesis and the corresponding lack of energy.

Carnitine deficiency has been linked to heart problems because the heart tissues prefer to utilise the fatty acids transferred by carnitine rather than other amino acids. Heart conditions have been helped with a high-carnitine diet.

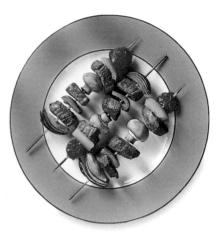

KEBABS WITH GRILLED VEGETABLES
Cut a thick piece of lean rump steak or lamb into cubes and skewer with pieces of pepper, onion, mushrooms and tomatoes. Grill for 15 minutes, turning occasionally. Beef is one of the richest sources of carnitine.

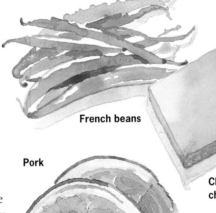

French beans

Pork

Cheddar cheese

Lamb chops

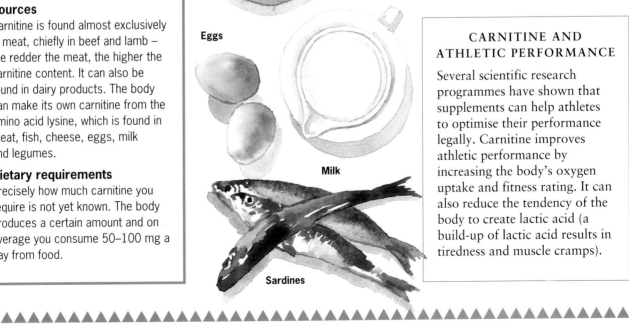

Eggs

Milk

Sardines

SOURCES AND REQUIREMENTS

Sources
Carnitine is found almost exclusively in meat, chiefly in beef and lamb – the redder the meat, the higher the carnitine content. It can also be found in dairy products. The body can make its own carnitine from the amino acid lysine, which is found in meat, fish, cheese, eggs, milk and legumes.

Dietary requirements
Precisely how much carnitine you require is not yet known. The body produces a certain amount and on average you consume 50–100 mg a day from food.

CARNITINE AND ATHLETIC PERFORMANCE

Several scientific research programmes have shown that supplements can help athletes to optimise their performance legally. Carnitine improves athletic performance by increasing the body's oxygen uptake and fitness rating. It can also reduce the tendency of the body to create lactic acid (a build-up of lactic acid results in tiredness and muscle cramps).

▼▼▼▼▼▼▼▼▼▼▼▼▼▼▼▼▼▼▼▼▼▼▼▼▼▼▼▼▼▼▼▼▼▼▼▼

Iron

Iron is an essential part of the proteins haemoglobin and myoglobin which transport oxygen in the red blood cells and muscles. It is also a vital component of many of the body's enzyme systems.

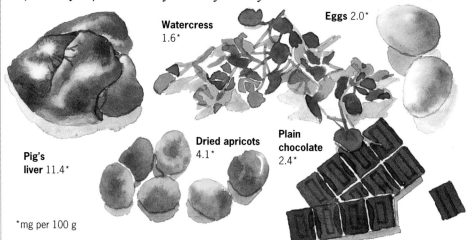

Watercress 1.6*

Eggs 2.0*

Dried apricots 4.1*

Plain chocolate 2.4*

Pig's liver 11.4*

*mg per 100 g

FACTORS THAT AFFECT IRON ABSORPTION

Tea and coffee taken with meals inhibit the amount of iron that can be absorbed. Studies have shown that it is best to wait for at least 1½ hours after a meal before having tea or coffee.

The phytate content of food also inhibits iron absorption. Phytate or phytic acid is found in wholegrain cereals, nuts and pulses. It binds with several minerals, such as iron, calcium, magnesium and zinc, during digestion and prevents them from being absorbed. Phytate is removed with the bran when white flour is produced.

There is also the weight factor. Although spinach contains nearly half as much iron as beef, at least ten times as much would have to be eaten for the same amount of iron.

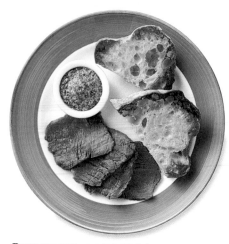

BRUSCHETTA WITH COLD ROAST BEEF
Lightly toast slices of ciabatta bread. Rub each slice with garlic and brush with virgin olive oil. Return to the grill for a minute and serve hot with thinly sliced, cold roast beef, rich in iron.

A recent report on iron by the British Nutrition Foundation claimed that 19 per cent of the world's population is iron deficient – a condition which compromises an individual's capacity to work and may, if untreated, cause delayed mental development in young children. Iron deficiency can cause a range of problems, mostly linked to anaemia (see page 136). The symptoms of anaemia include tiredness, sore tongue, cracks at the corners of the mouth and difficulty swallowing.

Iron deficiency is common in both Britain and the United States. Studies in Britain have found that about 25 per cent of pre-school children are iron deficient. Children with anaemia can suffer from learning difficulties and may have impaired physical development. Pregnant women and those with heavy periods, strict vegetarians and people who have a poor diet are also particularly at risk from deficiency.

Iron absorption from food and the availability of iron to the body is

SOURCES AND REQUIREMENTS

Sources
Rich sources are red meat, eggs and dried fruit. Poor sources include milk products, and it is important that babies eat solids from around six months of age as their foetal iron stores will have been depleted.

Dietary requirements
An average person needs around 10–15 mg daily.

affected by many dietary factors. Breast-fed infants absorb about 50 per cent of the iron in breast milk, but absorption from milk formulae is only about 10 per cent. Iron in meat is in a more available form and about 20–40 per cent is absorbed, but iron from vegetables and eggs is poorly absorbed and only about 5–20 per cent is available to be digested by humans.

▲▲▲▲▲▲▲▲▲▲▲▲▲▲▲▲▲▲▲▲▲▲▲▲▲▲▲▲▲▲▲▲▲▲▲▲

Tryptophan

Tryptophan is an essential amino acid which is needed in the daily diet for growth and repair. It is also known to be a mood enhancer and is important for the relief of stress, anxiety and depression.

If your diet contains sufficient vitamin B_6, tryptophan is converted to niacin and serotonin, a brain regulator or neurotransmitter. In the brain, serotonin induces sleepiness and sedation, promoting relaxation and the alleviation of stress.

However, getting high levels of tryptophan into the brain is not as easy as simply eating plenty of tryptophan-rich foods. Foods rich in tryptophan are proteins which are high in other amino acids, competing for the same entry point into the brain. Eating a high-protein diet actually reduces the amount of serotonin that reaches the brain. A high-carbohydrate diet will have a better effect on serotonin levels.

Tryptophan has been used in the treatment of depression and PMS, although research has not been conclusive in proving that tryptophan supplementation increases brain serotonin levels and improves mood.

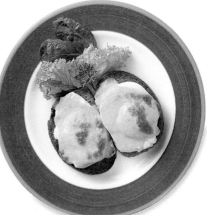

EGGS BENEDICT
Poach two eggs and lightly toast some bread. Make a hollandaise sauce by gently heating an egg yolk, half a tablespoon of water and a teaspoon of lemon juice until the mixture thickens slightly. Add 25 g (1 oz) butter, stirring in a little at a time. When creamy, pour over the poached eggs and brown quickly under a hot grill.

*mg per 100 g

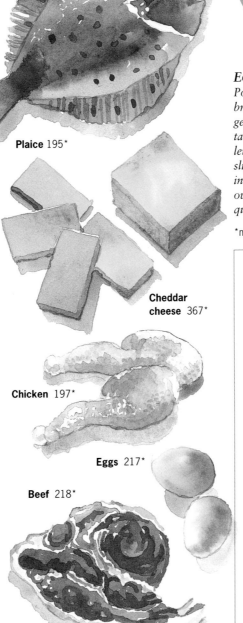

Plaice 195*

Cheddar cheese 367*

Chicken 197*

Eggs 217*

Beef 218*

SOURCES AND REQUIREMENTS

Sources
Tryptophan is available in most protein foods, although a high-carbohydrate diet is better for tryptophan absorption.

Dietary requirements
As yet, there are no recommended daily amounts.

TYROSINE

Tyrosine, like tryptophan, is an amino acid which is essential for the synthesis of adrenaline, noradrenaline, thyroid hormones and the brown pigment melanin. It is found in all food proteins and becomes raised in the plasma in relation to other amino acids after a high-protein meal. It has been suggested that this might have an effect on the production of neurotransmitters like noradrenaline and dopamine. Research has shown that some depressed people have low levels of tyrosine. When given tyrosine supplements, it is thought that neurotransmitter production is enhanced and mood improves.

Zinc

Zinc is fast becoming recognised as a very important nutrient for energy balance. It is involved either directly or indirectly in a wide range of metabolic processes which affect energy levels.

Many studies have shown zinc to be very important in maintaining the immune system. A Canadian research team in 1992 gave a dose of zinc to a group of elderly people. Those who received the supplement had only half the number of days troubled by acute infections and half the amount of antibiotics compared with those who did not. Also, some had evidence of mild nutritional deficiencies that cleared up.

Another study showed that taking a zinc supplement regularly during the period of a cold, starting within 24 hours of the first symptoms, significantly reduced (by almost half) the duration of symptoms.

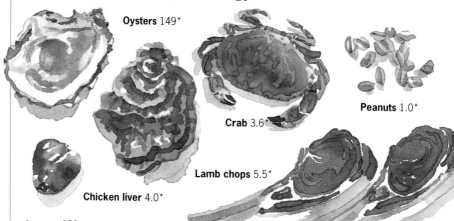

Oysters 149*

Crab 3.6*

Peanuts 1.0*

Lamb chops 5.5*

Chicken liver 4.0*

*mg per 100 g

Zinc is involved in the major metabolic pathways contributing to the metabolism of proteins, carbohydrates, fats and energy. Zinc helps tissue renewal and is involved in some of the enzymatic reactions necessary for the normal oil gland function of the skin.

Zinc research has progressed greatly through the study of an hereditary absorption defect in infants, known as acrodermatitis enteropathica. This condition occurs only in formula-fed babies; breast milk provides available zinc.

Deficiency symptoms include slow growth, infertility, hair loss, skin problems, diarrhoea, immune deficiencies, impaired senses and poor wound healing. Zinc deficiency can easily be detected by the presence of two or more white spots on your fingernails.

Studies have shown that a deficiency of zinc affects muscle strength and endurance. Exercise can increase the body's requirement for zinc; taking a supplement can reduce

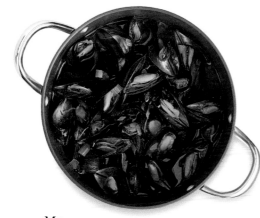

MOULES MARINIERE
Fry a chopped onion in a tablespoon of olive oil with a chopped stick of celery and a few crushed cloves of garlic. Add a pound of mussels in their shells, a pint of boiling water, chopped parsley and 2 tablespoons of white wine. Bring to the boil, cover and leave to simmer for 10 minutes. Serve in bowls with french bread. Seafood is a good source of zinc.

SOURCES AND REQUIREMENTS

Sources
By far the best dietary source of zinc is oysters. Other good sources are other seafood, red meat, nuts and seeds, eggs and wholegrain cereals. White flour is a poor source of zinc.

Dietary requirements
An adult woman needs 7 mg of zinc every day, a man needs 9 mg.

the damaging effect of extreme exercise on the immune system.

The amount of zinc absorbed from the diet varies greatly from 14 to 41 per cent as a number of factors affect zinc availability. Zinc in foods of plant origin is generally less available than from animal sources. The amount of phytate in the diet – present in wholemeal products – has been shown to affect absorption.

Coenzyme Q10

Coenzyme Q10, or ubiquinone, was first discovered in the late 1950s in the United States and was identified as a critical component in the production of energy within cells. Its effect decreases with age.

Coenzyme Q10 (coQ10) can be obtained from certain foods in the diet, or made within the body from two amino acids together with vitamins B and C. Dietary sources include most nutritious animal and vegetarian foods. Supplements are needed to achieve very high levels, although they are expensive and may be difficult to obtain.

CoQ10 can be regarded as the spark plug that ignites the fuel in the mitochondria and so produces energy. A deficiency of the coenzyme results in a reduction in energy and a slowing of metabolic processes.

Levels of coQ10 fall with age and in certain diseases. For example, heart patients may have low levels, with an increase occurring when supplements are taken.

*mg per 100 g

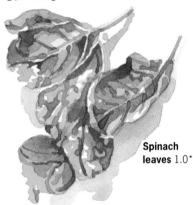

Spinach leaves 1.0*

Soya oil 9.2*

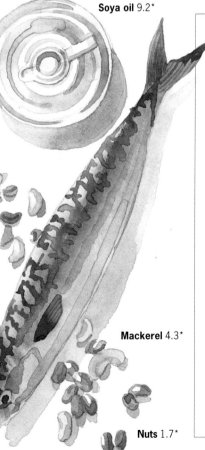

Mackerel 4.3*

Nuts 1.7*

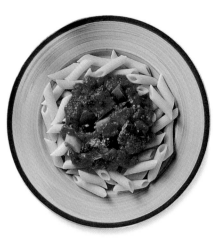

SARDINE AND OLIVE PASTA BAKE
Fry a chopped onion and pepper until soft and add a tin of chopped tomatoes, a tin of sardines in tomato sauce, some mixed herbs and halved black olives. Blend the mixture thoroughly, chopping the sardines, and serve liberally on a bed of freshly cooked pasta.

SOURCES AND REQUIREMENTS

Sources
Almost everything we eat contains various forms of coQ10. Good sources include soya products, nuts and seeds, leafy green vegetables, and oily fish such as tuna, trout and sardines.

Recommended intake
The recommended daily allowance has not been determined. In the light of experimental studies and findings, however, some scientists state that the daily requirement lies between 10 and 30 mg.

COENZYME Q10 AND AGEING

As we get older, our ability to ward off infection and diseases, such as cancer and arthritis, decreases. This decline is related to the strength of the immune system. Experiments carried out on mice have shown that coenzyme Q10 decreases with age; with supplementation an increase in life span occurred due to a healthier immune system. There is also a large amount of documented evidence that coQ10 has a positive effect on a number of illnesses associated with ageing, including heart disease, periodontitis and high blood pressure. Body tissue levels of coQ10 depend both on the dietary intake and the amount made within the body.

Magnesium

Magnesium helps to maintain the electrical balance of the body's tissues and is thought to be of particular importance in preventing energy problems. Some cases of fatigue can be alleviated by a high magnesium diet.

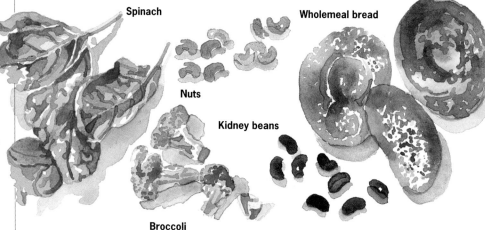

Spinach

Wholemeal bread

Nuts

Kidney beans

Broccoli

MAGNESIUM AS A FATIGUE CURE

The link between magnesium and fatigue was first discovered in the 1970s, when a group of medics in France began to prescribe magnesium supplements to people suffering from spasmophilia, which has similar symptoms to magnesium deficiency – aching, twitching muscles with headaches and mental disturbances. A team of doctors in Southampton found in the 1980s that giving magnesium supplements to chronic fatigue patients whose magnesium levels were below normal made an improvement in 80 per cent of cases. While further research has been unable to prove a conclusive link between energy levels and magnesium, it is often used to help to relieve chronic fatigue when deficiency seems to be a factor.

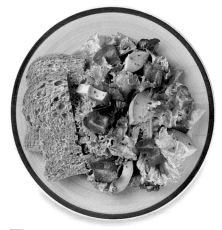

Warm bacon and avocado salad
Chop and fry two rashers of bacon in a small amount of olive oil. Toss them over a mixed salad with avocado. Serve with wholemeal bread.

Magnesium is vital for the effective action of many enzymes, so a lack can disrupt the operation of the body's nerves and muscles leading to poor functioning of the major organs, particularly the liver. Because magnesium is stored in the body in large quantities, however, deficiencies are rare. Where they do occur most cases are the result of digestive disorders, other illness, severe weight loss, alcoholism, or persistent diarrhoea and vomiting. Some drugs, such as diuretics, can cause deficiency and are a leading cause of magnesium troubles with elderly people.

Because so many body functions are reliant on magnesium, a deficiency may show itself in a variety of ways. A reduction in muscle efficiency is common, often associated with muscle fatigue, twitches and spasms. Personality changes, apathy, anorexia and other nervous disorders may also occur.

Supplements can restore magnesium levels, and boost energy

SOURCES AND REQUIREMENTS

Sources
Magnesium is widespread in foods, particularly green vegetables, as it is an essential constituent of chlorophyll which is necessary for photosynthesis.

Dietary requirements
The recommended intake of magnesium has been suggested to be 270 mg per day.

levels in previously deficient patients. They are also beneficial for blood sugar control, and can rebalance temporary reductions in blood sugar which can cause low energy. However, there are many energy problems that cannot be treated with extra magnesium; supplements seem to work best when they are used to rebalance already low levels of the mineral.

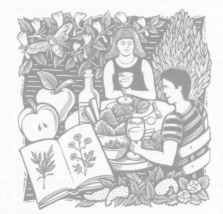

CHAPTER 5

A VITAL MIND AND BODY

Energising both your mind and body is key to improving your overall health and well-being. Through regular physical exercise you can increase the efficiency of your body at producing energy and boost your mobility and vitality. On a different level, practising relaxation and stress reduction techniques can improve your mental energy and your ability to cope with life's ups and downs.

REGULAR EXERCISE FOR ENERGY

Regular exercise can make dramatic improvements to your energy levels, improving blood flow, body functioning and oxygen supply, and refreshing your mental attitude.

The more active a person is, the more energy they will have for life. The body and mind need energy for repair and rejuvenation – it is essential in order to deal with the stresses and strains of normal life. A healthy body will have sufficient energy not only to keep itself in good repair, but also to cope with the additional energy demands of work and recreation. As soon as energy levels drop, the body will be less able to look after itself, and so less able to create energy, leading to a downward spiral of fatigue and poor health. Regular exercise will help to prevent you from falling into this kind of negative spiral by keeping your energy levels up.

OXYGEN AND ENERGY

Breathing in oxygen is essential to human existence – so much so that our bodies give us dramatic warning signs when supplies are inadequate. For example, if you exercise so strenuously that your body has insufficient oxygen to supply demand, you may experience severe muscle cramps that prevent you continuing the exercise. Similarly, if your brain is inadequately supplied, you may feel confused, dizzy and even lose consciousness. The efficiency of your oxygen supply depends on the efficiency of your cardiovascular system, and regular aerobic exercise is the only way to strengthen the heart and lungs.

Aerobic exercise includes any physical activity that demands the transportation of large amounts of oxygen to the working muscles via the blood for sustained periods. Running, cycling, swimming, dancing, aerobics and brisk walking all require such sustained muscle activity. If

continued for at least 12 minutes at a time they will raise your pulse rate and provide effective aerobic exercise. By contrast, activities such as weightlifting or sprinting require a short burst of energy and utilise existing supplies of carbohydrate in the body without the use of oxygen. This is known as anaerobic respiration, and can only be sustained for a limited time span before the muscle stops functioning.

Both aerobic and anaerobic exercise have health benefits, but it is aerobic that improves the body's cardiovascular functioning. Regular aerobic exercise of over 20 minutes three times a week is advised for boosting your body's ability to create and access energy when you need it.

Oxygen and the brain

During an exercise session the body will experience increased blood flow, promoting the transport of oxygen, the elimination of toxins, and the removal of stress, all of which promote a rise in available energy. The increased blood flow improves the supply of oxygen to the brain, which aids

FULL DRIVE AHEAD
Taking exercise can be an ideal way to focus on a different aspect of your abilities and refresh yourself to face everyday challenges.

healthy brain functioning. Laboratory research tests have shown that even though the brain makes up only 2 per cent of the body's total weight, it utilises 20 per cent of its available oxygen. Migraine headaches, as well as fatigue and a loss of concentration, can be the result of a lack of oxygenated blood in the brain.

MORE ACTIVE, MORE ENERGISED

Interestingly, vigorous physical or mental exercise can actually make you feel more energised rather than fatigued. This is because during physical exertion hormones known as endorphins are released into the blood from the brain. These act like a painkiller, reducing stress and pain and inducing a feeling of well-being. They are released so that the body or mind can continue to exert itself. If you exercise for a long time, for instance in a marathon, endorphins are produced to counteract the pain and fatigue in the muscles.

However, even moderate exercise can raise the level of endorphins, improving your mental outlook and reducing stress, one of the most significant energy drainers. The exercise–stress link has been proven by

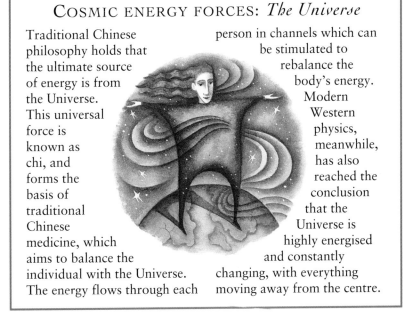

COSMIC ENERGY FORCES: *The Universe*

Traditional Chinese philosophy holds that the ultimate source of energy is from the Universe. This universal force is known as chi, and forms the basis of traditional Chinese medicine, which aims to balance the individual with the Universe. The energy flows through each person in channels which can be stimulated to rebalance the body's energy. Modern Western physics, meanwhile, has also reached the conclusion that the Universe is highly energised and constantly changing, with everything moving away from the centre.

a number of studies. For example, in the 1980s Herbert de Vries at the University of Southern California conducted an experiment with stressed and fatigued patients. He gave half of the group tranquillisers and the other half performed physical exercise every

continued on page 116

BREATHING EXERCISE

Emotions are intricately linked to breathing, probably due to neurochemical reactions between the body and mind. When you cry, your physical reaction is to catch your breath and breathe rapidly and deeply. An angry person breathes quickly, building up aggression and fuelling the body for physical action. You can help to relieve tension by breathing deeply but calmly.

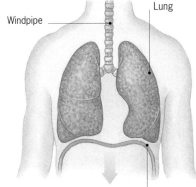

Windpipe

Lung

INSPIRATION | Diaphragm

1 When you take a deep breath, or inhale, your diaphragm moves down and your chest moves outwards as your lungs fill with air. Hold your breath for a few moments and feel the expanse of your lungs.

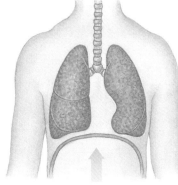

EXPIRATION

2 Expiring involves the upward movement of the diaphragm and the chest moves inwards. Practise breathing deeply for a few minutes, holding yourself upright for better air movement.

EXERCISE FOR A BETTER BODY

Physical exercise can help to energise your body in a number of ways. It can:

▶ *Improve the functioning of organs, especially the heart and lungs.*

▶ *Improve blood circulation.*

▶ *Increase the energy content of every cell in the body.*

▶ *Help to cleanse the body through improving the functioning of the lymphatic system.*

▶ *Help to reduce physical and emotional stress.*

▶ *Reduce excess adrenaline.*

A Home Work-out

Every morning when you get out of bed, put aside five or ten minutes to warm your body up and get the blood flowing properly. It will wake you up, helping you to feel great and topped up with energy for the rest of the day.

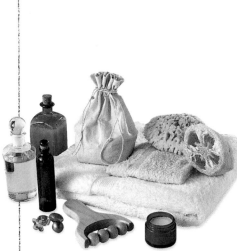

STRETCHING OUT IN THE BATH
After your home work out, take a soothing bath to enhance the relaxing qualities of exercise and rest.

These stretching exercises can be performed on your own at home at any time of day. They will take from 5–20 minutes, depending on how long you want to spend on each exercise. You may want to add your own exercises, or adapt these to your own level of fitness and flexibility.

There is no need to hurry, although you should ensure that your heartbeat is raised sufficiently to pump the blood around your body at a faster speed than normal. This will improve your body's ability to transfer oxygen and food to the cells and then convert them into energy.

1 *From a standing position, take a giant step forwards, keeping your hands on your hips for support. Lean into the step and hold for a few seconds. Return to standing position, then step forwards with the other leg. Repeat 8 times on each side.*

2 *Lie on your back with your knees bent and feet flat on the floor. Put your right hand behind your head and reach out with your left hand to touch your right knee. Relax back to lying position. Repeat 8 times on each side.*

Hold the position for a few seconds before relaxing

Back should be straight and upright

3 *Still lying on your back, put both hands behind your head and lift your legs so that your thighs are at right angles to your body, and your calves are parallel to the floor. Now raise your head, neck and shoulders off the ground, hold for a few seconds, and then relax back to the floor. Repeat 8 times.*

Keep your calves at a right angle to your thighs

Feet should be pointing forwards

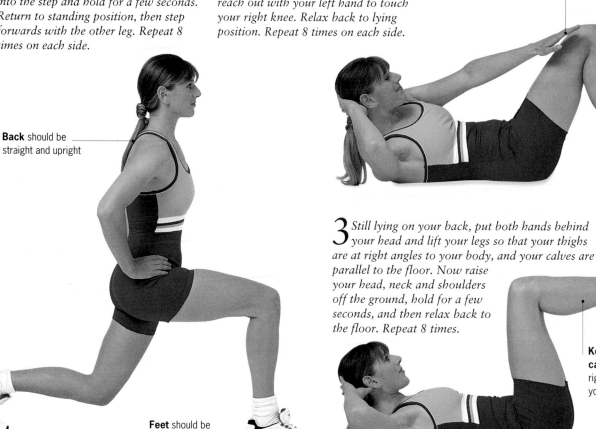

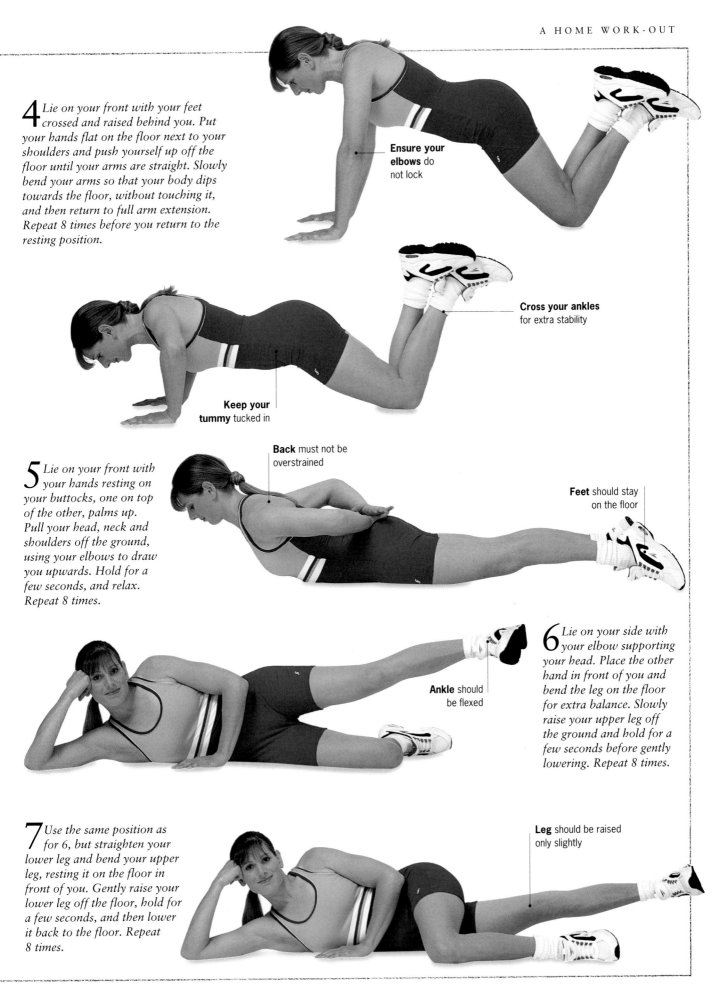

4 *Lie on your front with your feet crossed and raised behind you. Put your hands flat on the floor next to your shoulders and push yourself up off the floor until your arms are straight. Slowly bend your arms so that your body dips towards the floor, without touching it, and then return to full arm extension. Repeat 8 times before you return to the resting position.*

Ensure your elbows do not lock

Cross your ankles for extra stability

Keep your tummy tucked in

Back must not be overstrained

5 *Lie on your front with your hands resting on your buttocks, one on top of the other, palms up. Pull your head, neck and shoulders off the ground, using your elbows to draw you upwards. Hold for a few seconds, and relax. Repeat 8 times.*

Feet should stay on the floor

Ankle should be flexed

6 *Lie on your side with your elbow supporting your head. Place the other hand in front of you and bend the leg on the floor for extra balance. Slowly raise your upper leg off the ground and hold for a few seconds before gently lowering. Repeat 8 times.*

7 *Use the same position as for 6, but straighten your lower leg and bend your upper leg, resting it on the floor in front of you. Gently raise your lower leg off the floor, hold for a few seconds, and then lower it back to the floor. Repeat 8 times.*

Leg should be raised only slightly

day. From the results he discovered that as little as a 15-minute walk every day is more relaxing and efficient in dealing with stress than any course of tranquillisers.

STRETCHING

As with all forms of exercise, stretching is a vital warm-up, allowing your body to adjust to the strain of physical exercise. However, stretching also provides energy benefits. It can help to realign your skeletal structure, release tension from muscles and relax your joints, leaving you ready for action and exertion. In addition, it makes you feel good, liberating you from the confines of your normal movement and allowing you to release the pressures and anxieties that have been holding you back.

GETTING INTO EXERCISE

Although the health benefits of regular exercise are irrefutable, it can still be difficult to change a sedentary lifestyle to a more active

DID YOU KNOW?

An important element of Chinese Taoist philosophy is to 'embrace the uncarved block of wood', meaning that you must see yourself as a new entity which has the potential to be carved into any number of forms. Do not try to fit into a mould, restricting yourself with rules and regulations, or be led by others. Let your natural energy flow freely and tell you which path is best for you.

one. It may be especially difficult if you are suffering from fatigue. Some people find that a change is best achieved by fairly dramatic means such as signing up for a year's membership of a local gym. Other people, however, find it easier to make a gentle adaptation from their current lifestyle. If you remember that any form of physical activity is helpful you should be

ASHTANGA VINYASA YOGA

'Yoga' means union and it is the union of mind, body and spirit that yoga aims to achieve. Regular practice of yoga will result in improved flexibility, strength, posture, respiration, increased energy, tranquillity and motivation.

Ashtanga vinyasa yoga is a method of yoga that has been in existence for some 1500 years. It was rediscovered in 1930 and is now practised worldwide. Ashtanga vinyasa yoga aims to unite physical (*hatha*) and mental (*raja*) yoga through a variety of postures, breathing and concentration. Each posture (*asana*) should ideally be held for as long as possible to enhance muscular strength and suppleness, although for beginners this may not be advised in the initial stages. The focus is firstly towards alignment of the body to improve physical balance. If a body is in natural alignment this will improve posture and decrease muscular tension. Attention is then given to specific breathing patterns, or *pranayama*, designed to stimulate the energy flow, or *prana*, in the body.

SURYANAMASKAR – SALUTE TO THE SUN
An Ashtanga vinyasa yoga session will usually start with the Suryanamaskar – a basic exercise to harness energy. Move gradually through the positions in a flowing movement. The exercise is supposed to be done several times, quite quickly, so that you feel puffed out by the end. Take care if you have back problems.

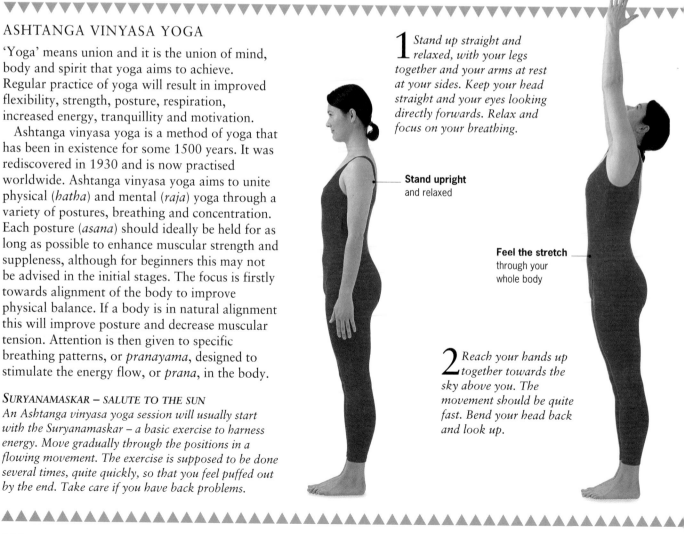

1 *Stand up straight and relaxed, with your legs together and your arms at rest at your sides. Keep your head straight and your eyes looking directly forwards. Relax and focus on your breathing.*

Stand upright and relaxed

Feel the stretch through your whole body

2 *Reach your hands up together towards the sky above you. The movement should be quite fast. Bend your head back and look up.*

able to integrate more activity into the things you already do. For example, simply deciding to take a walk in your lunch hour rather than sitting in the staff canteen can make a difference if you gradually increase both the frequency of your walks and your speed. Exercise in the middle of the day can also give you a much needed energy boost for the rest of the day. Walking up stairs rather than taking a lift or escalator can also boost your health. Instead of sitting on the sofa and watching the television, you can do some simple exercises to enhance your fitness and flexibility. Try a few leg lifts, head rotations and arm stretches. Don't think of how you can avoid as much physical effort as possible, think of how you can maximise your exercise opportunities.

EASTERN EXERCISE TRADITIONS

Eastern systems of health have long recognised that exercise is integral to energy levels. In fact health systems such as Ayurveda

SEX FOR ENERGY AND HEALTH

Sex is an excellent energy enhancer, and can also relax you thoroughly. Not only is it a highly effective form of physical exercise, using a large range of muscles, but it is also a great mood enhancer, helping you to feel good.

► *Aerobic exercise benefits can improve your heart and lungs.*

► *For women, regular sex increases oestrogen levels, improving skin, hair and menstrual imbalances.*

► *Endorphins are released by the pituitary gland, lifting mood and countering stress.*

► *Touch is emotionally soothing.*

► *Muscles are relaxed through the sexual act and physical contact.*

► *Boosting the immune system, regular sex has been found to counter breast cancer development.*

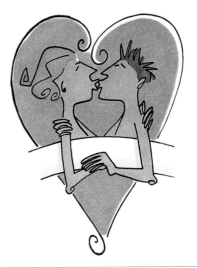

3 *Bend right down from your hips, keeping your legs straight and together. Try to touch your legs with your head, although this may be difficult at first.*

Bend your knees if you cannot reach

4 *Keeping your hands on the floor – bend your knees if you cannot reach – transfer your weight onto your palms, look up and prepare to jump or step back.*

5 *Without moving your hands, jump or step back, then gently lower your body, keeping your elbows in. Bend your arms so that your shoulders are raised just above the floor as if to do a press-up.*

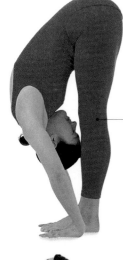

Keep your arms straight and hands flat on the floor

6 *Roll forwards onto the front of your toes and push your upper body forwards and up by straightening your arms. Curl your back and look upwards.*

7 *Using your hips to push up, roll back onto the soles of your feet and straighten your back, with your arms straight and your hands on the floor in front of you.*

Back and shoulders must be straight and stretched out

(see page 48) and therapies such as yoga or t'ai chi and chi kung use exercise as a core feature of a complete approach to improving and balancing energy flow in the body.

Chi kung is divided into two general categories: a tranquil or meditative aspect where the emphasis is on concentration, visualisation and breathing; and dynamic chi kung based on activity. Each aspect of the therapy is equally important in bringing about a proper flow of life energy in the body, often focusing on restoring energy balance (see also pages 120–1). A number of experiments have indicated that chi kung benefits both the mind and the body. A research project conducted at the Shanghai Institute of Hypertension found that chi kung appeared to reduce the risk of cardiovascular disease and that this was due both to its impact on circulation and its relaxing effect. The mixture of physical exercise with uplifting meditative movements makes chi kung a remarkable therapeutic experience.

MIND–BODY LINK

Researchers have recently learnt that the emotions and the body are intricately linked by neuropeptides – a group of chemicals that transport messages between the brain and the body. Neuropeptides are responsible for telling you to feel thirsty or hungry, for stimulating good feelings or creating the sensation of pleasure. It has been found that breathing deeply – such as during breathing exercises or meditation – can cause a flood of emotions. This is because the part of the brain stem responsible for breathing is thickly endowed with neuropeptides and neuropeptide receptors which cause a heightened, positive and vital mood. Focusing on your breathing can therefore lift mood and help to balance your energies.

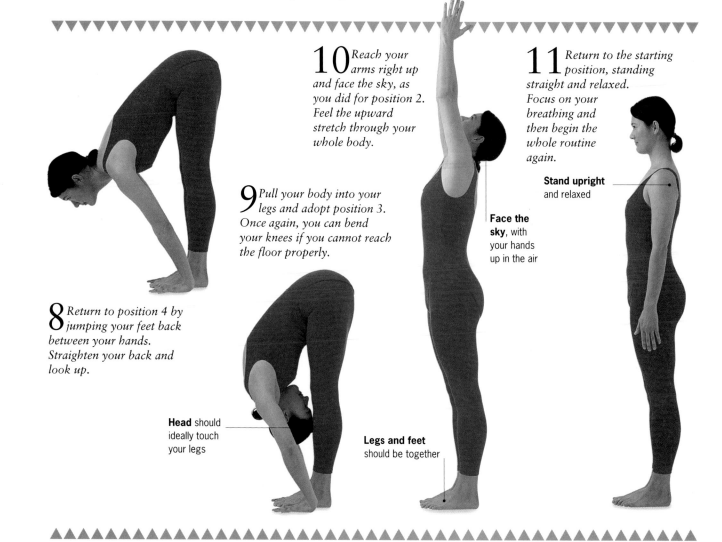

8 *Return to position 4 by jumping your feet back between your hands. Straighten your back and look up.*

9 *Pull your body into your legs and adopt position 3. Once again, you can bend your knees if you cannot reach the floor properly.*

Head should ideally touch your legs

10 *Reach your arms right up and face the sky, as you did for position 2. Feel the upward stretch through your whole body.*

Face the sky, with your hands up in the air

Legs and feet should be together

11 *Return to the starting position, standing straight and relaxed. Focus on your breathing and then begin the whole routine again.*

Stand upright and relaxed

ENERGY AND YOUR EMOTIONS

Both positive and negative emotions can sap your energy. After any extreme emotion, the body's energy reserves are lowered, and rest and recuperation are required.

When you experience an extreme emotion – good or bad – your body calls upon its ability to produce the 'emergency' hormones which help you to cope with the need of the moment. The instant an extreme emotion is recognised, the body sets off its arousal system. The adrenal glands produce adrenaline, noradrenaline and corticosteroid hormones which begin to surge around the body, causing the muscles to tighten, the heart to beat faster, and the breathing to quicken, and reducing the blood supply to the skin.

This energises the body, enabling it to respond quickly to the emotion. However, this emotional surge draws heavily upon the body's reserves, which must be restored. Normally, the body can do this through sleep and the digestion of food, but sometimes the hormones do not know when to switch off and you remain on a 'high' for far longer than necessary. This can cause insomnia and a loss of appetite, or a craving for sugary foods, which are stimulants that can lead to adrenal gland exhaustion.

continued on page 122

EMOTIONS AND YOUR ENERGY BODYCLOCK

Your energy levels rise and fall throughout the day depending on your emotions, stresses and periods of rest and relaxation. When the energy-building emotions are not in balance with the energy-draining emotions, an energy deficit will result, leaving you tired and in need of rest and recuperation. Periods of great stress need plenty of relaxation to refresh energy levels and rebalance the negative effects of the stress.

A TYPICAL DAY
Every day brings a variety of emotional challenges. Making sure that you balance your emotional energies can help you to stay on top of daily stresses.

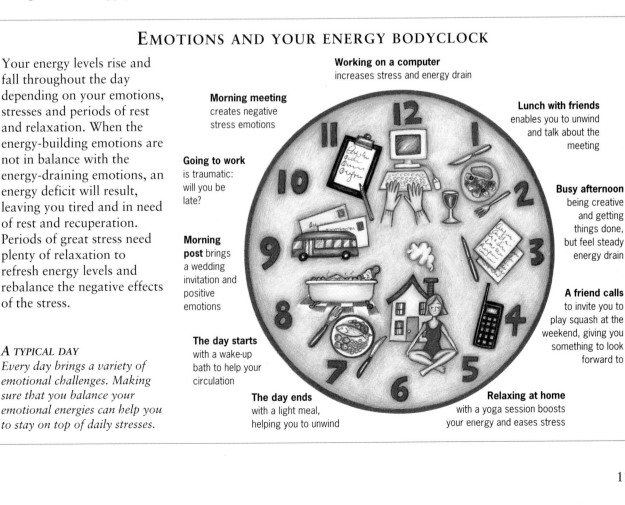

Working on a computer
increases stress and energy drain

Morning meeting
creates negative
stress emotions

Lunch with friends
enables you to unwind
and talk about the
meeting

Going to work
is traumatic:
will you be
late?

Busy afternoon
being creative
and getting
things done,
but feel steady
energy drain

**Morning
post** brings
a wedding
invitation and
positive
emotions

A friend calls
to invite you to
play squash at the
weekend, giving you
something to look
forward to

The day starts
with a wake-up
bath to help your
circulation

The day ends
with a light meal,
helping you to unwind

Relaxing at home
with a yoga session boosts
your energy and eases stress

119

The Chi Kung Teacher

Chi kung is the cultivation of internal energy – the vital breath of life that gives us the wherewithal to function healthily. Dance movements, often imitating the movements of animals and embodying their powers, are used to restore positive energy.

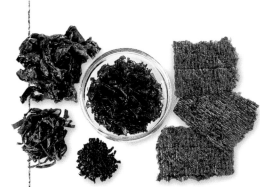

DAILY SEAWEED
Chi kung practitioners recommend eating one or two tablespoons of seaweed every day for good health. Seaweed can also be taken in tablet form.

DURING A CLASS
The moves are first demonstrated by the teacher, who then helps the class members through each aspect of the movement.

Chi kung is practised by performing specific movements in coordination with breathing and meditation techniques. The exercises aim to energise and rebalance the body, uniting body, mind and spirit in a natural, unrestricted way. Practising these energy exercises regularly can help you to find the energy to enjoy a happier, healthier and less restricted life.

What happens during a chi kung session?
A chi kung session takes place in silence to help the mind to focus completely on the exercises and the movement and restoration of energy. The teacher will lead a warm-up routine, including breathing exercises, posture adjustments and a variety of smooth-flowing exercises that gently loosen the joints and create body heat. The chi kung exercises are then taught, mostly step by step, with the teacher clearly demonstrating the exercises and giving explanations regarding what to focus on and specific details of each movement.

Because all the movements are performed at a very slow pace, it is possible to follow the teacher through some of the movements, and he or she will watch and correct your posture afterwards. You may be asked to retain a posture for several minutes, focusing your mind during this time on your breathing. Another element that may be incorporated is self-massage, which helps to stimulate the flow of chi through your body. If you are practising with a group of people it is usual to perform all the exercises in a circle.

What qualifications does a chi kung teacher have?
There are no official qualifications; length of practice and expertise are the most common indicators of a teacher's skill. In China, a committee of masters can qualify a person who is well practised in chi kung to become a master.

What are the benefits of chi kung?
Chi kung exercises can lead to remarkable improvements in your health as well as making you feel livelier and happier. The aim of a chi kung session is to relax, energise and

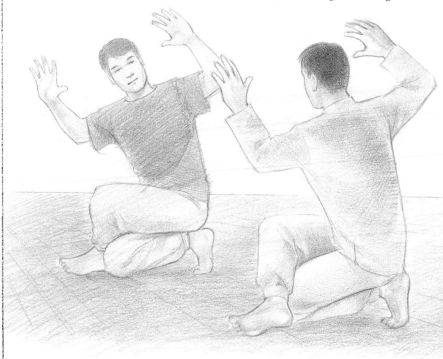

Origins

Elements of chi kung have been used for thousands of years. Ancient cave paintings in China depict dance moves imitating the characteristics of animals, which later became the more structured energy exercises incorporated into the Taoist spiritual tradition, which encourages harmony between the individual and the natural world. The Taoist Canon (a treatise of 1120 volumes) contains all the early texts of chi kung, which were subsequently influenced by Indian yoga and Tibetan Buddhism. Chi kung has continued to be practised up to the present day, although it was discouraged by the Chinese communist regime for much of the 20th century. Dr Qian Xue-sen, a scientist educated in the United States, returned to China during the Cultural Revolution (1966–76) and re-established the tradition.

restore balance to both your body and your mind. To achieve these benefits the session incorporates a variety of specific exercises, including stretching, breathing and mental exercises, which stimulate the flow of chi. According to the principles of traditional Chinese medicine, stagnant chi in the body is the chief cause of illness. Chi kung is designed to help the chi to circulate more efficiently and thus restock the body with fresh energy.

You should be able to feel the positive effects of chi kung even after the first session. One of the initial benefits is to feel a sense of calmness and a clarity of mind. In the long term, chi kung can improve your emotional health and stability, and it has also been known to help combat specific psychological and physical illnesses.

What are the 'Three Treasures' and how are they used?

Central to the philosophy of Taoism, from which chi kung derives, is the concept of the Three Treasures. The first of the Three Treasures is jing, which is both sexual energy and the germ of life. The second is chi, the omnipresent energy of life. The last is shen, which means 'stretch' and symbolises the subtle energy of the spirit, stretching up towards the Universe. These treasures have been likened to the energies of the mind, body and spirit; each is a crucial part of the whole and the idea is to refine jing to chi, refine chi to shen, and ultimately refine shen and return to the void. The void is a state of empty clear-mindedness – your original mind untouched by concepts or images – and this is the ultimate goal of practising chi kung. Chi kung uses movement to effect this transformation, aiming to help you to understand each state through breathing and physical awareness and balance.

WHAT YOU CAN DO AT HOME

Stand with your feet a little more than hip-width apart, and legs slightly bent at the knee. Feel your spine lengthen and come into alignment. Relax the shoulders and face muscles. Start to breathe deeply. Inhale through the nose, and focus on the breath going into the lower part of the stomach. Spread your arms out and imagine them as branches growing naturally into the outside world. Exhale and imagine your feet growing roots penetrating the earth, grounding you and giving you strength. Practise this for 5 minutes. This exercise is a good way to rejuvenate the body's circulation.

STANDING LIKE A TREE
This simple exercise can help to promote a sense of being 'rooted'. It can be helpful during moments of anxiety or trauma, or for general relaxation.

How can chi kung help with emotional problems?

Stress and anxiety build up when your emotions are suppressed in order to cope with everyday demands. Chi kung breathing exercises draw attention to your breath, which clears your mind and creates an awareness that allows you to tune in to how your inner self is feeling about your life and identify any problems. This is known as 'listening to the energy'. By freeing your deeper feelings, you will find your inner self less burdened and restored to emotional health.

Chi kung thus aims to resolve emotional issues, some of which you may not even know that you have. The stress relief will unburden your muscles and body, and slow your pulse and heartbeat, improving physical health and energy. The feeling of emotional calm and balance experienced with chi kung also has an invigorating effect, replenishing your energy and leaving you feeling refreshed.

Focus on your breath travelling right down to your navel

121

COSMIC ENERGY FORCES: *The Sun*

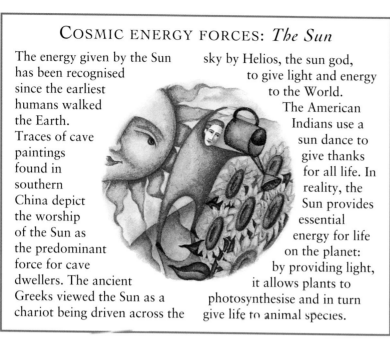

The energy given by the Sun has been recognised since the earliest humans walked the Earth. Traces of cave paintings found in southern China depict the worship of the Sun as the predominant force for cave dwellers. The ancient Greeks viewed the Sun as a chariot being driven across the sky by Helios, the sun god, to give light and energy to the World.

The American Indians use a sun dance to give thanks for all life. In reality, the Sun provides essential energy for life on the planet: by providing light, it allows plants to photosynthesise and in turn give life to animal species.

EMOTIONAL STRESSES AND ENERGY

Stress experts have categorised stress – including all the different kinds of mental, physical and emotional stresses – into three sequential phases: phase one harnesses the body's energy reserves, phase two utilises these reserves, and phase three drains them and leads to exhaustion. Emotional stress fits into phase three – and it drains the energy reserves more than any other form of stress, affecting physical and mental, as well as emotional reserves.

As your body struggles to cope with the demands of extreme emotions, 'unnecessary' emotions tend to be lost: your sense of humour and your talent for enjoying life disappear. Behavioural changes may also occur; for example, a once happy-go-lucky person can become quiet and withdrawn. You may not notice these changes in yourself, but others will. Motivation is reduced and tasks become harder to perform. Concentration is impaired and planned thinking becomes difficult. Anxiety about the inability to cope in all the different areas of life distresses the sufferer further. The end result is complete exhaustion – and when the body's energy reserves are exhausted, opportunistic illnesses occur.

The body's ability to protect itself and fight infection is governed by the immune system, which is directly controlled by the mind and the way that you are feeling emotionally. Negative emotions and thought patterns reduce the efficiency of the body's defence system because they drain energy that could otherwise be used to prevent illness. Studies carried out at the Common

THE THREE PHASES OF STRESS

Researchers have found that, faced with a stressful situation, the body uses energy in three sequential phases. The third phase is important since worrying about a past experience helps you to understand danger and prevent future stress. However, it can be extremely draining if you cannot relax properly. Try to review the crisis calmly and understand that the danger has passed and you are now safe.

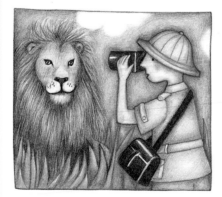

PREPARING ENERGY
Phase one is when you ready yourself, harnessing energy reserves. You sense the danger and your body is preparing for a 'fight or flight' reaction.

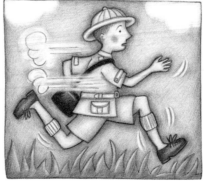

UTILISING ENERGY
Phase two is when you are utilising your energy reserves. Your body is working to its full potential to help you get through the situation.

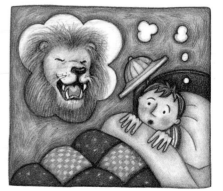

DRAINING ENERGY
Phase three is when stress continues and you are draining your energy. You may be out of danger, but your body and mind cannot calm down.

Clear Your Mind with

Standing Meditation

The single most important and widely practised form of chi kung is standing meditation. It aims to develop better alignment and balance, stronger legs and waist, deeper respiration, body awareness and a tranquil mind.

Start by practising for 5 minutes each day, spending equal amounts of time in each position. After a week, increase the time to 15 minutes a day; after three weeks you should be able to meditate for 20–40 minutes every day. Stand with the feet a little more than hip-width apart. The knees should be slightly bent. Try to achieve a natural alignment of the spine, free from tension. It can help if you imagine a thread pulling up from the base of your neck through the top of your head. Begin the exercise with your arms relaxed and slightly in front of your body.

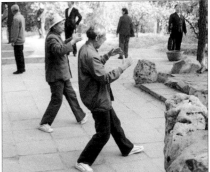

DAILY BREAK
Many Chinese people practise chi kung every day for health, often outdoors in squares or parks.

SIMPLE STANDING MEDITATION

Spend a minute or so simply focusing your attention on your body. Begin by focusing on your feet and work your way up through each part of your body, paying particular attention to the spine. Relax and free up any tension, feeling the contact of the floor.

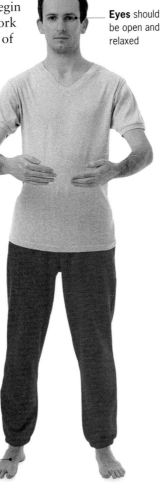

Eyes should be open and relaxed

Arms should be in a rounded position

Feet should be a little more than hip-width apart

Be aware of whatever presents itself in your consciousness, giving yourself permission to feel or think anything that you want

Hands may be raised to your head, but not above

Breathing should be completely natural, relaxed and from the diaphragm

1 *Bring your hands up in front of your abdomen, with both palms facing towards your body as if you are embracing a large, light-weight ball. Inhale slowly and move your hands upwards, palms facing the body, to your waistline and hold the position for a few seconds.*

2 *Raise your hands further up your body while inhaling, bringing them in towards your head and gently turning your palms around to face forwards. Hold for a few seconds, then slowly start to exhale and work your arms and hands down in front of you, palms towards your body. Repeat the whole exercise several times.*

Cold Unit at Oxford University showed that people who had suffered negative emotions during the previous six months were more likely to get colds than those who had good coping skills for negative emotions. In addition, the incidence of colds was significantly higher in people who were introverted, indicating that people who can call on good support mechanisms to share their negative life experiences are better able to handle the difficult emotions such experiences generate than those who hold them inside.

You should learn to use your energy wisely and build up a reserve for emergencies. You should also learn to recognise your physical and emotional thresholds and take preventative action before you deplete your energy reserves.

CHOOSING YOUR EMOTIONS

Most negative emotions and thoughts can be turned into positive ones, rechannelling energies into good actions. Some psychologists believe that we choose the emotions we experience. When we reach our threshold of endurance – which we, ourselves, set – we allow ourselves to 'go over the edge' and express our frustration. Where we set these limits can be 'reasonable', in that this is where most people would set their limits, or 'unreasonable', in that our reactions are extreme or inappropriate or brought about by irrational thinking.

How you react to a situation is up to you. If you don't like your job, change it. If, for various reasons, you can't, try to change it from within – speak to your boss, suggest alterations, or ask for a transfer to another department. It is important to remember that you always have an option.

Some negative emotions, when viewed from another perspective, can become positive. Anger does not have to be negative – it can serve as a trigger to do something positive about the situation that is making you angry. Envy can be transformed into admiration and become an inspiration. Anxiety can help us to recognise situations in which we need to learn better coping skills.

Feeling empowered is highly energising and motivating. The elation you get from achieving something positive cancels out

A FRIEND IN NEED

When friends or relatives are at a low ebb and perhaps do not know where to turn – or even why they feel so unhappy – you can give invaluable comfort. Even if you cannot help in practical ways, just listening allows the other person to share his or her problems and thus reduce stress and anxiety. If you need support, do not be afraid to ask friends or family to listen to your troubles; they are usually willing and able to help.

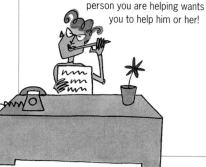

Listening is the most helpful thing you can do. Try to empathise with the person and attempt to understand what has triggered off such unhappiness.

Help or suggest help if you can. Perhaps you can offer a practical solution or provide the address of an organisation or professional advice body. Make sure the person you are helping wants you to help him or her!

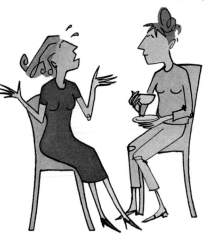

ASK QUESTIONS
After listening, try to ask some questions to help the other person focus on the problem. It may reveal aspects that had not previously been considered and give an opportunity to see the problem from a different angle.

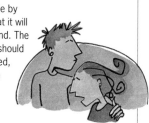

Comfort and console by telling the person that it will all be alright in the end. The value of comforting should not be underestimated, although it should be backed up with positive help if possible.

Support is important. Few crises disappear overnight – and emotional problems are no exception. Your role as friend is to provide long-term support. Visit and phone regularly. Be the type of friend you would want for yourself.

Avoid judgment, whatever the problem is, and especially avoid criticism. Professional counsellors aim to reveal to the sufferer ways in which they can help themselves. They never offer their own opinions, so neither should you.

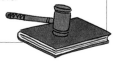

CASE STUDY

The Irritable Mother

Emotional problems can seriously drain your energy, especially if they are ignored or repressed. The result is that you will behave differently, often expressing your pent-up feelings through bitterness or anger. Giving yourself time to identify and acknowledge the causes of your distress, and talking these over with those close to you, can help you through the difficult times.

Roselyn is a full-time mother with two sons at school. Her husband has recently been promoted and frequently spends time away on business, leaving her on her own to look after the boys. Her mother died unexpectedly last year of leukaemia and she has found herself growing stoical about life, not admitting that her emotions are getting her down. She has been experiencing a general loss of energy, culminating in difficulties leaving the house. She is snapping at the children and her husband, blaming his absence for all her problems. She went to the doctor and had a series of tests for fatigue disorders, but no specific cause could be located. Her doctor suggested that she went to see a counsellor.

WHAT SHOULD ROSELYN DO?

Roselyn should go to a counsellor, who will talk with her about her life and lifestyle and how she feels about her family. Counselling could help Roselyn to root out the underlying cause of her irritability and unhappiness by allowing her to talk freely about her emotions and uncover deeper problems and anxieties. Facing her mother's death and allowing time for proper grieving should be a priority. Rather than snapping at her family, she must talk calmly to them about her needs, and they in turn should arrange to give her time and space to recover. The doctor may also prescribe a short course of antidepressants to help Roselyn cope with her unstable emotions.

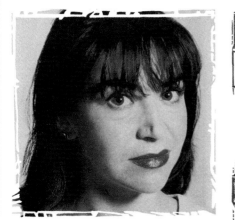

FAMILY
Family problems can build up if you do not openly discuss issues as they arise.

LIFESTYLE
Keeping going without taking proper rest can seriously damage your emotional and physical health.

DEPRESSION
Emotional problems such as depression can drain energy and create greater difficulties.

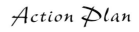

Action Plan

LIFESTYLE
Make time for self. Keeping too busy to face problems only allows them to build up inside.

DEPRESSION
Talk to a counsellor to help to identify and resolve the underlying causes of depression. Understanding and facing emotions is the first step to emotional health.

FAMILY
Talk to family and friends about worries and grief. Recognise that irritability and anger are counterproductive means of expression.

HOW THINGS TURNED OUT FOR ROSELYN

Roselyn's counselling helped her to accept the toll her mother's death was taking on her emotional and physical health. She became aware that she had alienated her husband as a result of his being away, and they spent time restoring their relationship. He adjusted his work schedule so that he could spend more time at home. She joined a local chi kung class which helped her to relax and restore her emotional and physical energy.

ORGANISE AND PRIORITISE

Whether at work or in your personal life, learning to organise and prioritise clears away confusions, allowing you to be more efficient.

▶ *Keep up to date with your filing, so you know where everything is and when it needs attention.*

▶ *Keep a wall calendar and diary. Look at it every day to check what you have to do.*

▶ *Keep a list. Write down everything you need to do and tick off those you have done.*

▶ *Prioritise your list. Categorise entries, marking those that are urgent.*

▶ *Don't use delaying tactics. Phone people you have to phone and leave personal calls for later.*

▶ *Learn how to say 'no'. Recognise your limits and don't take on what you can't do.*

▶ *Keep a set of accounts so you can see how much you are spending and how much you have.*

▶ *Learn to delegate. You do not have to do everything yourself.*

KEEPING IN TOUCH
Friendships are among the most rewarding parts of our lives, supporting us through the bad times and giving us another point of view.

negative feelings and beliefs that can be harmful. Taking charge of your life is one of the greatest energy boosts you can have.

YOUR SUPPORT MECHANISMS

Even the most self-sufficient of us can recognise the positive help that others can give us. There are times when it is unwise to fight your battles on your own and recognising when you could do with the help of friends, counsellors or spiritual guidance will help you through your problems.

Spiritual guidance

In times of emotional distress, many people feel a need for spiritual or religious support. Irrespective of religious doctrine, leaders of religious groups are trained in supporting those who need spiritual or emotional help. Religious beliefs can be very comforting in times of emotional upset, when the world ceases to make any sense. Many alternative therapies offer different spiritual philosophies which can refresh your outlook and help you to view the world from a different, and often healthier, angle.

Friendship

One of the greatest support systems you have is your friends and, because they are likely to be familiar with your circumstances, they may be able to offer useful and supportive advice. However, you should choose your confidante wisely. Choose someone who will listen, help and, above all, be able to keep a confidence. This may be someone other than your best friend or partner – it can be better to talk to someone who is not so involved and can see your problems from an objective standpoint.

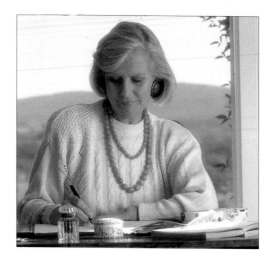

CHANGE YOUR LIFE

Change begets change – if you change one thing in your life you will find that other things change around it, providing you with a new direction and focus. Change is renewing and replenishing, providing you with the opportunity to fulfil yourself in new ways. Change can also be daunting, but if you make the changes gradually it will seem less intimidating.

Be positive about change. Pursue new interests or hobbies which provide you with mental and/or physical stimulation. Join a gym, a dance class or an evening course. Become a volunteer for a charity – help yourself through helping others.

Don't forget to challenge your brain, particularly if you do not work or are retired. Learn about literature, history or a new language, join a reading group or become an expert in something that interests you.

Counselling

Sometimes problems are deep rooted or very complex and require the skills of a counsellor. As opposed to therapists, counsellors are trained to ask questions and listen to you, helping you to sort out your own problems rather than making any judgments or diagnoses for you. In this way, counselling can give you insight into your feelings and empower you to solve your own problems. With the guidance of a counsellor, you can resolve inner conflicts and find practical solutions. If you feel that counselling sessions could help you, ask your doctor to refer you to a fully trained counsellor or contact the British Association of Counselling.

Energising therapies

There are a range of alternative therapies which can help you to revitalise your energy channels, removing stresses and pressures and releasing unwanted tension. Many of these rely on Eastern holistic philosophies (see page 48) which view energy as a universal force that flows through your body. Therapies such as t'ai chi, chi kung, Reiki and shiatsu aim to rebalance your energy, allowing your natural forces to work freely.

CHAPTER 6

SERIOUS CONDITIONS AND ILLNESSES

If you are lacking in energy for a prolonged period of time, you may have a more serious underlying condition. A number of conventional tests can identify specific illnesses, and various treatments can help to counter both the ailment and the lack of energy. Some energy disorders, however, benefit most from a more holistic lifestyle approach involving diet, exercise and stress reduction.

CONSULTING YOUR DOCTOR

Lack of energy is commonly associated with another underlying medical condition. Locating and treating debilitating conditions can restore your health and vitality.

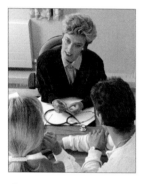

GO PREPARED
Before visiting the doctor make a brief list of all your symptoms so you do not forget to mention something during the consultation that may help with your diagnosis.

Most people feel tired and lacking in energy from time to time, and distinguishing when there is a particular or serious problem, rather than a 'bad day' or a temporary minor illness, can be difficult. Monitoring your health to gauge whether persistent fatigue has been nagging you for a few weeks or more is usually the best way to tell if there may be a more serious problem to consider.

Before you go to the doctor, you may find that you can alleviate the condition yourself by ensuring that you are eating properly (see Chapter 4) and following some of the basic health guidelines such as regular exercise. If, however, your fatigue lasts for more than two weeks and you cannot locate a direct cause, such as a common cold or lack of sleep, you should visit your doctor.

VISITING YOUR DOCTOR

Although fatigue can be caused by a number of problems – physical, emotional or psychological – physical disorders are usually the easiest to diagnose and treat. A visit to your doctor can help to reveal any underlying health disorders and provide treatment to restore your health.

Many studies have found that complaints of lack of energy are commonly caused by

WHAT CAN MEDICAL TESTS TELL YOU?

A number of tests may be carried out initially, such as a general observation, physical examination and blood and urine analyses, which can indicate possible problem areas. Further tests are used to locate more specific problems.

You may find yourself referred to a specialist clinic or hospital department for further tests and treatment.

FULL EXAMINATION
A thorough examination usually includes assessing the condition of your skin, hair, nails, tongue, eyes, ears, chest, abdomen, lymph glands, nervous system, heart, lung function, blood circulation and reproductive health.

▶ **NUTRITIONAL TESTS**
The blood can be tested for a wide range of nutrient deficiencies, including iron, vitamin B_{12}, folic acid, other B vitamins, magnesium and zinc.

▶ **URINE TEST**
A quick and easy test, urine can show up kidney, bladder and urethral disorders as well as blood sugar levels and diabetes.

▶ **INFECTION TESTS**
Immunoglobulin tests can monitor antibody levels and indicate hidden infections.

▶ **THYROID TEST**
If a patient has energy problems, the levels of the thyroid hormones in the blood are measured to find any imbalances.

▶ **BLOOD TEST**
Blood tests examine the numbers and shapes of blood cells and the nutrient levels in circulation to identify any dietary deficiencies, infections or diseases.

an underlying physiological disorder. For example, in 1980 Dr John D. Morrison, a doctor in the US, reviewed 176 patients with chronic fatigue. He found that 69 of the patients were suffering from minor or serious physical problems, including viral infections, heart, lung and thyroid disorders, arthritis and nutritional deficiencies.

In addition, he found that 21 patients were suffering from both physical and psychological problems. In 72 other cases, he diagnosed psychological problems as being the main cause of chronic fatigue. Other studies have found that blood abnormalities can play a major role, and thyroid disorders can be the cause of a number of complaints.

If your doctor does not find any apparent physical problems which may be causing your lack of energy, it may mean that your problem is either physical, but cannot be located, or it is psychological. As Dr Morrison's study reveals, psychological problems can be the underlying cause of a great number of fatigue problems, or can occur alongside physical problems to compound the debilitating effects of illness.

Medical experts believe that some fatigue patients are suffering from a psychosomatic reaction to major emotional upheavals or upsets, such as the death of a loved one, or pressure to achieve more than they are capable of. In these cases, the doctor may recommend psychological treatment such as psychotherapy or analysis. However, many psychological problems can themselves be the result of physical disorders and must not be assumed to be the only or primary cause of fatigue.

WHAT MAY BE CAUSING YOUR FATIGUE

Fatigue is the symptom of a number of disorders, illnesses and conditions, and one of the hardest tasks that your doctor faces is finding which single or combined cause is resulting in your lack of energy. It is important to go to your doctor if you suffer from any of the following symptoms for a prolonged or recurrent period. The table is a guide only, and is no substitute for a doctor's examination.

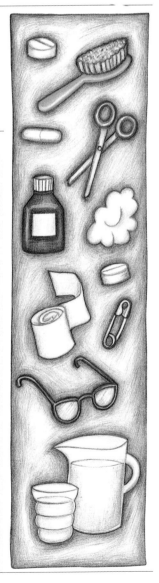

SYMPTOMS	POSSIBLE CAUSES
Have you experienced sudden tiredness recently?	Infections
Do you feel particularly tired when getting up in the morning?	Hypoglycaemia, insomnia or other sleeping disorders
Do you feel tiredness with a headache or dizziness?	High or low blood pressure, hypoglycaemia
Do you have tiredness associated with digestive troubles?	Enzyme deficiency, disturbed gut flora
Do you feel ill if you miss a meal?	Hypoglycaemia
Is your tongue red, sore or fissured?	Anaemia
Have you suffered from a loss of hair on your head, a dryness of skin or chilliness?	Thyroid gland deficiency
Have you noticed a deterioration of eyesight, a great thirst or poor wound healing?	Diabetes, nutritional deficiency
Do you get breathless easily?	Heart or lung problems
Have you had a recent head injury?	Nervous system shock
Do you bruise easily?	Anaemia, nutritional deficiency
Do you have swelling of ankles and feet?	Heart and circulation disorder
Have you been suffering from recurrent infections?	Depression of immune system, diabetes, thyroid deficiency

High or Low Blood Pressure

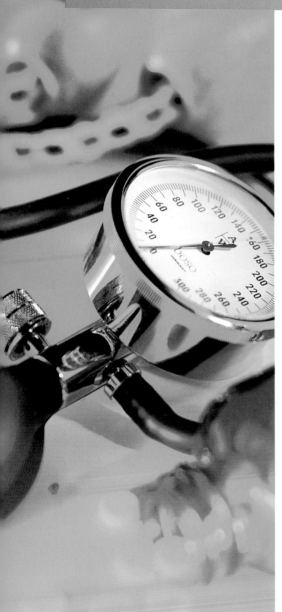

Blood pressure problems are relatively common and can lead to serious heart and lung disorders if left untreated. Following a balanced diet and managing your stress levels will help to protect against blood pressure problems.

THE PROBLEM

Blood pressure is an indication of the power of the heartbeat and the amount of resistance in the blood circulation. A reasonable pressure must be sustained to ensure that sufficient blood reaches the brain and the limbs. But if the pressure falls low or is consistently too high it leads to a range of physical disorders.

Blood pressure is recorded as two sets of numbers which measure the pressure in a column of mercury transmitted from a cuff wound round the arm. The higher figure (systolic pressure) represents the pressure during the heart's contraction phase and the lower figure (diastolic pressure) is the relaxation phase.

Normal blood pressure for an adult is below 140/90, and slightly lower in children. Blood pressure varies a little according to activity, but if it becomes consistently high it is known as high blood pressure (hypertension). At the other end of the scale, low blood pressure (hypotension) occurs when the systolic pressure drops below 100.

High blood pressure may be caused by a deeper problem, such as disease of the heart, kidneys, lungs, liver or blood vessels. In the majority of cases, however, there is no apparent cause for the high blood pressure (essential hypertension). Persistent high blood pressure can be a serious threat to health, with a greater risk of strokes or heart attacks.

BLOOD PRESSURE FACTORS

A number of factors, especially when combined, are thought to contribute to hypertension including:

▶ *Being overweight.*

▶ *Having too much salt, sugar, caffeine and alcohol in the diet.*

▶ *Smoking.*

▶ *Over-competitive personality.*

▶ *Prolonged stress.*

▶ *Pregnancy may cause high blood pressure in some cases.*

▶ *A lack of physical exercise.*

Low blood pressure is marked by light headedness when changing position quickly and coldness of the extremities. It is mostly a less severe disorder than hypertension, but may indicate a weakness of the adrenal glands, anaemia and poor nourishment. A sudden dramatic drop in blood pressure as a result of injury or disease is called clinical shock and is a life-threatening condition requiring emergency aid.

Both high and low blood pressure may be responsible for tiredness but they rarely show obvious symptoms until a blood pressure test is carried out during a routine medical examination. Once detected they should be monitored regularly and regulated with professional guidance on diet and lifestyle, supported by other treatments where necessary.

SYMPTOMS

▶ Light headedness and dizziness in low blood pressure

▶ Fainting in low blood pressure

▶ Cold extremities in low blood pressure

▶ Fatigue in both high and low blood pressure

▶ Headaches in high blood pressure

DIETARY MEASURES

Dietary advice forms the cornerstone of hypertension management. Some problems will improve merely by excluding salt from the diet.

Reduce sugar
High sugar intake may cause sodium retention and contribute to high blood pressure in some individuals.

Avoid stimulants
Both caffeine and nicotine cause a temporary increase in blood pressure and should be avoided.

Cut down on fat
Saturated fats, for example from meat and dairy produce, may lead to a build-up of fatty deposits in the arteries (see pages 85–86) and must be strictly limited, especially fat from red meat. In a recent study, vegetarians were found to have significantly lower blood pressure compared to non-vegetarians.

Complementary approaches
For hypertension, a naturopath may recommend fresh juices or lacto-fermented juices as good sources of essential minerals, such as potassium and magnesium, which help to balance blood pressure. Short fasts on juices and raw food dietary regimens under naturopathic supervision are effective in reducing blood pressure. In a recent trial, a dietary regimen of raw fruits and vegetables was found to be as effective as conventional drugs in reducing blood pressure. Take a glass of grape and celery juice twice daily for 20 days, and then stop taking it for seven days before repeating the process. Supplements of vitamin E may be helpful, along with potassium, calcium and magnesium.

For hypotension, a naturopath may provide nutrients to support the thyroid and adrenal glands and maintain blood sugar levels.

HERBAL TREATMENT

Some herbs have the effect of restoring the balance in both hypertension and hypotension, for example hawthorn berries (*Crataegus oxyacantha*). Herbs with reputed blood pressure lowering properties include: yarrow (*Achillea millefolium*), garlic (*Allium sativum*), and skullcap (*Scutellaria lateriflora*).

People with low blood pressure tend to be slender in build and easily fatigued. Suitable herbal remedies may need to be prescribed to help to compensate for these susceptibilities. In particular, tonic measures may be suggested to sustain the cardiac output and support the tone of blood vessels as well as glands such as the adrenals. Ginseng (*Panax ginseng*), prickly ash (*Xanthoxylum americanum*), and broom tops (*Sarothamnus scoperius*) may be considered.

ACUPRESSURE POINTS

The powerful relaxation effects of acupressure are believed to account for its success in treating high blood pressure. This traditional Chinese technique of energy rebalancing through pressure relieves stress and enhances well-being by opening the energy channels at specific points where blockages occur. Apply firm but gentle pressure to the following acupressure points with a fingertip or thumb for two or three minutes at a time. You may also use dispersed pressure by gently massaging the whole area.

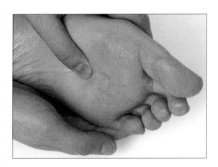

KIDNEY 1
This point is on the bottom of the foot, in the central depression one-third of the way down the foot.

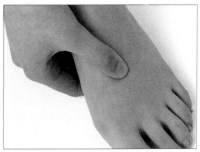

LIVER 3
This point is on the top of the foot, in the angle between the long bones leading to the first and second toe.

HYDROTHERAPY

There is a range of hydrotherapy techniques that can be used to treat low blood pressure.

▶ *Turn your morning shower cold for a few seconds before you get out. This stimulates the faster movement of blood around the system and is particularly good for the skin and the hair.*

▶ *Use alternate hot and cold foot baths to encourage better blood flow in the arteries. Spend a few minutes in each before you change.*

▶ *Placing an icepack or a cold, damp flannel against the back of your neck will force the blood to pump faster around your body.*

▶ *Go for a swim. Even if you are not very good, it is great for your blood pressure, as well as your all-round health. Try to do some stretching exercises in the water to keep active and flexible.*

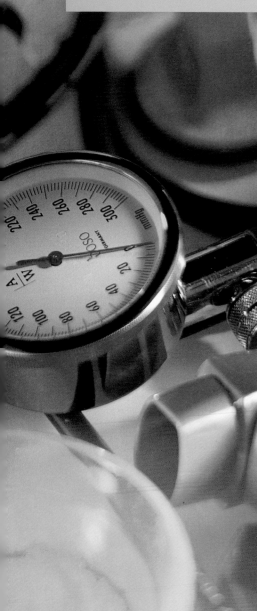

Heart and Artery Disease

Heart and artery disease severely restricts the lives of many people, draining energy and preventing healthy activity. Heart conditions claim thousands of lives every year, and yet are often preventable by simple changes in diet and lifestyle.

THE PROBLEM

Heart and artery disease is caused by fatty deposits, or plaques, which build up on the walls of the arteries, causing narrowing and blockage – a condition known as atherosclerosis. The heart needs a constant supply of oxygen, glucose sugar and other nutrients which it receives through its own network of blood vessels, called coronary arteries. If these arteries are narrowed by fatty plaques, the blood flow to the heart muscle is restricted. The heart can then no longer cope with physical exertion, even walking upstairs may be difficult. Physical effort causes severe chest pain – a condition called angina pectoris – and can limit a sufferer's ability to lead a normal life.

Once a coronary artery is blocked completely, so that no blood can get through, some of the heart muscle dies causing a heart attack. The severity of the heart attack depends on the amount of heart muscle that has been damaged, but it is always serious and often fatal. Heart disease is believed to be the most common cause of death in middle age, and the second most common killer overall, after cancer.

AGE CONCERN
As you get older, the chances of suffering from a heart or an artery disorder increase greatly, so exercise and dietary regimes should be adopted to lower the risk.

CAUSES OF HEART AND ARTERY DISEASE

The build-up of fatty deposits around the heart and artery system is encouraged by several factors:

▶ *A diet high in saturated and hydrogenated fats, found in foods such as meat, dairy products, pies, sausages and convenience meals.*

▶ *Some people have naturally high cholesterol levels.*

▶ *After the menopause, women are more prone to heart problems.*

▶ *Smoking.*

▶ *An inactive lifestyle.*

▶ *A diet that is high in salt, which also collects in the artery system.*

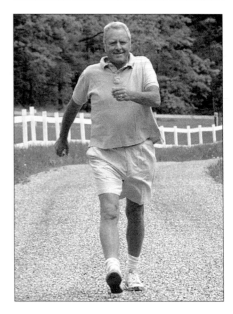

SYMPTOMS

▶ Tiredness during and after physical exertion
▶ General fatigue
▶ Pains in the chest
▶ Irregular heartbeat or heart palpitations
▶ Blueness of the skin caused by a lack of oxygen in the blood
▶ Can cause faintness after physical exertion

DEALING WITH A HEART ATTACK

Heart attack is very common and it is important to know what to do if it occurs to someone near you. The symptoms often start as a mild ache that is often confused with indigestion. This may turn into moderate or severe pain in the centre of the chest that radiates down the left arm or up to the jaw.

Always seek medical advice if you, or a person you know, have unexplained abdominal or chest pains that are not relieved by mild over-the-counter medication. Chest or abdominal pain that is severe, persistent or recurrent always requires immediate medical attention. Other common symptoms include sweating, paleness, faintness, rapid and shallow breathing, and a sense of impending danger.

The first priority in a heart attack is to dial 999 and ask for an ambulance. Loosen the casualty's clothing and tilt the head back to open the airway and make it easier for the casualty to breathe. Give the casualty a soluble 300 mg aspirin tablet and ask him or her to chew it slowly, without water. If the casualty suffers from angina, he or she may have glyceryl trinitrate (GTN) as tablets or inhaler. Give one tablet or two puffs of inhaler. If the casualty loses consciousness place in the recovery position. If breathing stops apply emergency resuscitation, if you have been taught the technique.

FOOD SUPPLEMENTS

Antioxidants such as folic acid and vitamin E have proved effective at preventing heart and artery disease when taken as supplements. In several studies, increased consumption of antioxidant vitamins in the diet or as supplements reduced the risk of heart disease by up to 40 per cent in men and 25 per cent in women.

Another popular heart supplement is coenzyme Q10. This nutrient is necessary for cellular energy production and is particularly important for aiding the heart muscle. However, supplements can be expensive and hard to find.

REDUCING THE RISK OF HEART AND ARTERY DISEASE

Diet and lifestyle are the main underlying causes of heart and artery disease. Major changes here can go a long way towards reducing your risk of heart attack. It can also make a great difference to your all-round health and energy levels.

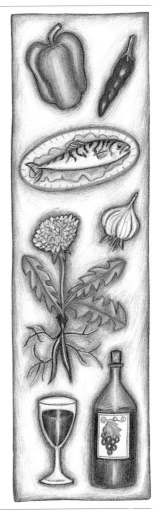

EAT MORE FRUIT AND VEGETABLES

Eat plenty of brightly coloured fruit and vegetables, which contain the antioxidants beta-carotene and vitamin C. These protect the heart against free radicals – unstable molecules produced by metabolic processes and pollution – which encourage fat build-up.

KEEP ACTIVE

An inactive lifestyle is a major cause of heart disease. Stay active and, in particular, take regular aerobic exercise such as brisk walking, running, cycling or swimming for 20–30 minutes three times a week. This strengthens heart muscle and inhibits fat build-up.

EAT MORE FIBRE

Soluble fibre, found in fruit, vegetables, peas, beans and oat bran reduces blood cholesterol levels.

HORMONE REPLACEMENT

If you are post-menopausal, hormone replacement therapy (HRT) helps to protect against heart disease.

EAT OILY FISH

Include plenty of oily fish, such as salmon and tuna, in your diet. These types of fish contain omega-3 fish oils which can strengthen the heart, lower blood pressure and lower blood cholesterol levels.

SPICES OF LIFE

Include more fresh ginger, garlic and cayenne pepper in the diet. Ginger and garlic reduce the stickiness of the blood and reduce clotting. Cayenne pepper is effective for widening blood vessels.

MANAGE STRESS

Control your stress levels. Stress leads to raised blood pressure and increases the risk of heart and artery disease. Relaxation exercises can help.

MODERATE DRINKING

Drink alcohol – especially red wine – in moderation. This helps to raise levels of a substance called high density lipoprotein which protects the heart tissue.

HAVE AN ASPIRIN

Consider taking half an aspirin tablet each day to reduce the stickiness of the blood platelets and so prevent blood clots. Discuss this with your doctor.

HERBAL REMEDIES

Ginkgo biloba is thought to increase blood flow to the heart muscle and reduce blood clotting. Dandelion root can reduce high cholesterol levels.

Lung Disorders

The lungs are at risk from various diseases that may be avoided by taking preventive measures. This is particularly important in the case of cigarette smoke and pollution, which damage the lungs and make them vulnerable to infection and cancer.

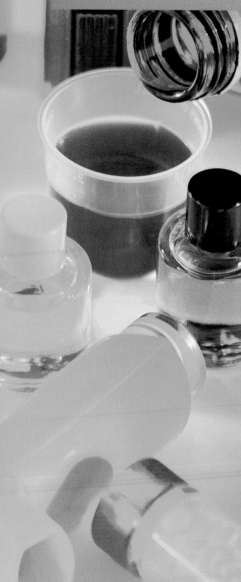

THE PROBLEMS

As you breathe, your lungs take in particles in the air such as dust, fumes, microorganisms and allergens (causes of allergy). As a result, the lungs are under constant threat from toxic substances and diseases.

The lungs are linked with the heart, so heart disorders (see pages 132–3) can cause lung problems.

Infection is the most common lung disorder, including coughs. Severe infection leads to acute bronchitis – the inflammation of the airways (bronchi) branching off the windpipe.

If a serious viral or bacterial infection spreads to the surrounding lung tissue it causes pneumonia. If it spreads to the membranes lining and surrounding the lungs (pleura) it causes pleurisy. Both require urgent medical attention.

Acute bronchitis stops once an infection is over. But another form, chronic bronchitis, can last indefinitely. It is usually caused by cigarette smoke, polluted air, or exposure to dust or fumes at work – which irritate the bronchi. Chronic bronchitis that causes extensive damage to lung tissue can lead to emphysema. Here, the groups of air sacs (alveoli) that absorb oxygen break down. This condition is incurable, other than by transplant.

Asthma is often caused by an allergy to airborne particles, such as house dust, pollen, pet hairs and feathers, chemical sprays, and certain foods. It leads to contraction of the muscles of the bronchi and increased production of mucus in the lungs. Asthma is usually a chronic condition that occurs as periodic attacks. Sufferers need to manage the condition by avoiding known irritants and using inhalant drugs to clear congestion.

Certain jobs carry a risk of occupational lung disorders and it is important to take precautions. Pneumoconiosis can develop from coal dust, asbestosis from asbestos fibres, silicosis from stone dust, and byssinosis from textile fibres. These can lead to emphysema and, along with smoking, are common causes of lung cancer.

CAUSES OF LUNG PROBLEMS

The most common causes of lung disorders are airborne pollutants, infections and irritants:

▶ *Virus or bacterial infection.*

▶ *Pollutants, such as dust and soot.*

▶ *Chemical fumes.*

▶ *Airborne allergens, such as pollen.*

▶ *Inhaling cigarette smoke, or other drugs.*

▶ *Smoky atmospheres.*

▶ *Heart and artery disease.*

▶ *High blood pressure.*

SYMPTOMS

▶ Persistent cough with thick yellow, green or grey phlegm

▶ Persistent coughing, wheezing or shortness of breath

▶ Difficulty breathing

▶ Blood in the phlegm

▶ Chest pain

▶ A blue tinge to the skin

▶ A high temperature or chills

▶ Swollen legs

AVOIDING LUNG DISORDERS

The lungs are quickly irritated by atmospheres that are too dry or too wet. Living in damp homes and areas with high rainfall raises the risk of developing chronic bronchitis and emphysema. Deal with damp problems promptly and ensure good heating and ventilation.

Modern central heating and air conditioning systems in homes and offices create very dry, dusty atmospheres. This irritates the lining of the lungs and increases the risk of colds and flu, leading to coughs and asthma attacks. Dry air also thickens mucus, making it more difficult to cough up. You can improve air quality by ensuring adequate ventilation. Place bowls of water near heaters to humidify the air.

Asthma sufferers should try to identify allergens and avoid them where possible. Mould spores, house dust, and animal dander – particles from pet hairs and feathers – are common allergens. Regular cleaning prevents a build-up of mould, dust and dander, and covering mattresses in polythene reduces house dust mites. Putting pillows in a freezer for a few hours kills dust mites. Refrain from smoking and avoid smoke-filled areas. Always wear a suitable mask if exposed to fumes or dust particles.

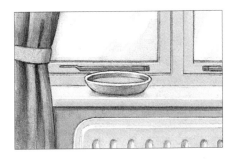

HUMIDIFIER
Keeping the atmosphere of a room moist can help to ease lung problems. Placing a dish of water over a radiator is an inexpensive and easy way of humidifying your home.

SUPPLEMENTS

Supplements may be taken to improve immunity and functioning.

▶ *During the winter, or when you have an active infection, take 500 mg of vitamin C twice a day. It is more effective with bioflavonoids, such as rutin.*

▶ *Zinc supplements aid the immune system. Sucking a zinc lozenge at regular intervals also helps to prevent viral infections spreading to the lungs.*

▶ *Vitamin A is quickly destroyed by cigarette smoke and atmospheric pollution. Vitamin A supplements, such as fish liver oil capsules, may be advisable. Too much vitamin A is harmful, however, so avoid exceeding the recommended dosage.*

▶ *Iodine, found in seaweed supplements, reduces the incidence of lung disorders.*

TREATING LUNG DISORDERS

For many lung disorders avoiding the underlying causes – such as cigarette smoke, or polluted atmospheres, or specific allergens – is the only realistic approach. Most infections will run their course naturally; rest in dry, warm conditions, and a healthy diet are usually sufficient treatment. More serious infections require medical attention. Cough medicines are of limited use. They come in two types: expectorants, for chesty coughs, loosen the mucus so that it can be more easily coughed up; cough suppressants soothe dry, irritating coughs. Never use a cough suppressant for a chesty cough; it can cause the mucus to build up in the lungs and may lead to more serious lung disorders.

An effective measure is steam inhalation. Pour hot water into a bowl and inhale the vapour. This loosens the mucus and opens the airways. You can try adding a few drops of menthol, eucalyptus or peppermint oil.

Regular aerobic exercise strengthens the heart and lungs and helps to reduce the risk of lung disorders. Brisk walking, cycling, jogging or swimming for at least 20 minutes three times a week is effective. Even those suffering from chronic bronchitis find that regular gentle exercise improves lung function and reduces feelings of breathlessness. Start with a few minutes and slowly build up as you feel stronger. Stop at once if you feel very breathless or have chest pains.

You can greatly improve lung capacity by regular deep breathing exercises, drawing air from the abdomen, rather than taking rapid, shallow breaths.

NUTRITIONAL ADVICE

Vitamin C is vital for a healthy immune system, so ensure your diet includes plenty of citrus fruits and green leafy vegetables. Vitamin A aids repair of the cells, especially the mucus lining of the lungs. To ensure you have an adequate intake include foods such as fish oils, dairy products, spinach, liver, carrots, apricots and margarine.

Naturopaths recommend a diet high in fresh fruit and vegetables (65 per cent) and low in protein (10 per cent) and fat (5 per cent). Complex carbohydrates, preferably wholegrain or unrefined forms, should make up the rest of the diet. Reduce your intake of refined sugar, including sweets, cakes and manufactured soft drinks, which depress the immune system.

Anaemia

Many people suffer from anaemia, which reduces the body's ability to produce energy and leads to deep fatigue. Making sure that you get the right nutrients can prevent anaemia, and many therapies stress the use of supplements to cover deficiencies.

THE PROBLEM

If you complain of persistent tiredness, one of the first things your doctor may do is to test your blood for anaemia. Anaemia is a deficiency of either the red blood corpuscles or the haemoglobin which they carry, or both. It diminishes the ability of the blood to carry oxygen to the tissues. The symptoms of anaemia grow worse as the deficiency of haemoglobin becomes more serious. Early symptoms include pallor, fatigue, lethargy, easy bruising and headaches, followed by difficulty breathing and dizziness. Further symptoms include heart problems, jaundice and heart attack.

Anaemia is most frequently caused by a deficiency of the nutrients needed for the formation of blood, particularly iron. Vitamins C and B_{12} and folic acid are also important. The disorder may also be caused by a digestive problem preventing the nutrients from being absorbed into the blood.

Anaemia can be the result of a blood defect, particularly due to a problem with the haemoglobin, the oxygen-carrying factor in the blood. It can also be caused by disturbances of the production of the red blood corpuscles which carry the haemoglobin, or because of a loss of the red blood cells due to haemorrhage or destruction.

Although less common, some anaemia cases require specialist medical attention and need blood transfusion, bone marrow transplant, spleen treatment, drug therapy or injections. However, the majority of cases can be treated with dietary measures and supplements.

CAUSES OF ANAEMIA

Many people have slight anaemia, particularly women due to blood loss at menstruation. Common causes include:

► *Insufficient iron in the diet.*

► *Deficiencies in vitamins C, B_{12} and folic acid.*

► *Inability to absorb nutrients.*

► *A large loss of blood due to haemorrhage or injury.*

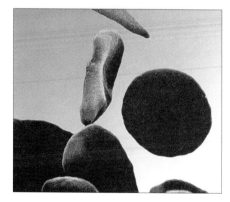

ANAEMIC BLOOD CELL
Anaemia occurs when the haemoglobin in the red blood cells is unable to absorb oxygen. This may be caused by a variety of different conditions or defects.

SYMPTOMS

► Tiredness and lethargy

► Pale complexion, sometimes with a green or blue tinge

► Headaches

► Poor skin, hair and nail condition

► Loss of appetite

► Breathlessness after physical exertion

► Dizziness and inability to concentrate

► Difficulty breathing

DIETARY MEASURES

A number of nutrients are essential for the formation of healthy red blood corpuscles and to ensure adequate levels of the minerals they carry. Iron, copper, B complex vitamins, including folic acid, and vitamin C all play an important role in blood formation and a varied and healthy diet should provide these.

The richest food sources of iron are wholegrain cereals, such as rice and wholemeal bread, red meat, liver, egg yolk, cauliflower, green peppers, raisins, dried apricots, and green leafy vegetables. Although spinach has a high iron content it also has high levels of oxalic acid which binds with the iron preventing its absorption. Many of these foods are also excellent sources of other nutrients needed for blood formation, such as copper, calcium, folic acid and vitamin C.

Protein from offal, such as liver and kidneys, is considered to be an important source of iron and vitamin B_{12}, although vegetarian alternatives include eggs, cheese, nuts, seeds and soya products. Fortified foods or supplements may be beneficial.

Vegetables that have been through a lacto-fermentation process or have been made into a juice are known to be good for blood disorders because they are easier to digest. The process breaks down the indigestible cellulose component making the food an excellent and palatable source of nutrients. Lacto-fermented beetroot juice is reputedly of particular benefit for blood-related disorders.

Some disorders can affect the ability of the stomach lining to produce a substance called intrinsic factor, which is necessary for the absorption of vitamin B_{12}. Other intestinal problems can have the same effect and there may be a need to provide supplementary vitamins.

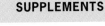

SUPPLEMENTS

In certain cases, digestive enzymes or preparations made from plant sources, such as pineapple and pawpaw, may also be needed to improve the digestive functions.

▶ *Iron deficiency is the primary cause of anaemia and supplements can improve a number of cases. Take 15 mg iron in tablet form twice a day.*

▶ *Vitamin C improves the uptake of iron and ensures that the folic acid remains active in the digestive system. Take up to 500 mg daily.*

▶ *Vitamin B complexes are also important. Vitamins B_6, B_{12} and folic acid are all necessary for blood production and functioning. A reputable B complex multi-vitamin should meet your needs, but you should seek the advice of your doctor or a dietitian if you have any queries.*

IRON-RICH SNACKS

Many foods that are rich in iron also make tasty and nutritious snacks and so are easily included in the diet. It is important not to focus only on iron, however, since other trace elements and vitamins, notably vitamin C and zinc, also play a large role in blood haemoglobin levels and can affect the amount of iron taken up by the body. Eating a variety of foods and avoiding processed foods are the main dietary objectives.

Wholemeal bread and pasta are high in iron, although the iron is not easily absorbed into the human body, and so other sources are also necessary to top up your stores of iron.

BOOSTING IRON
Nuts and dried fruit make an easy and portable snack. Egg and cress sandwiches, a dark green salad or a bean soup are also high in iron.

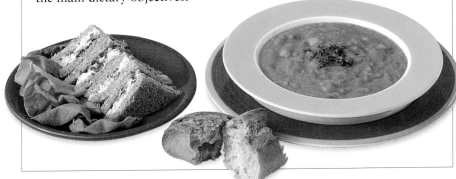

RESEARCH ON IRON DEFICIENCIES

The most well-known study was conducted in the US by Dr Ernest Beutler in 1960. After giving 29 women who complained of fatigue a complete physical examination, he found that 22 had low iron stores, and 7 were normal. He gave them all placebo tablets for three months, followed by iron supplement tablets for three months. He then asked them which tablets had made them feel less fatigued. Although the response was mixed from the 7 normal women, out of the 22 who had low iron stores 15 said that the iron gave them more energy, 5 preferred the placebo and 2 had no preference. The test therefore showed that giving iron to iron-deficient women can help with certain fatigue problems.

Adrenal Gland Problems

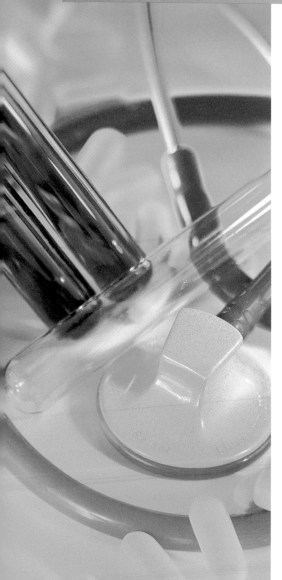

The adrenal glands provide the body with essential hormones that stimulate activity and energy. Problems with these glands lead to energy disorders, leaving the body unable to convert food into energy or cope with routine physical tasks.

THE PROBLEMS

The two adrenal glands are located on top of each kidney. They can be divided into two distinct parts which are responsible for producing very different hormones. The outer part, called the adrenal cortex, produces corticosteroid hormones and small amounts of the male hormone androgen (in both men and women). The inner part, called the adrenal medulla, produces the hormones adrenaline and noradrenaline.

Corticosteroid hormones have a range of important effects in the body. One of these hormones, aldosterone, helps to regulate fluid levels in the body and so plays an important part in controlling blood pressure. Another hormone, hydrocortisone (or cortisol), controls the way the body uses nutrients, especially proteins, fats and carbohydrates, and helps the body to recover from stress. This hormone, together with hydrocortisone, also affects the immune system and reduces inflammation. Androgens play an important part in female sex drive and a lesser part in male sex drive and sexual characteristics.

Adrenaline and noradrenaline are mainly released during times of stress. Their job is to prepare the body for physical activity by speeding the heart and breathing rate and diverting blood to the muscles.

As the adrenal hormones have such varied effects, disorders of the glands

ADRENAL GLAND FACTORS

The exact origin of adrenal gland problems is often difficult to locate since disorders can be prompted by a number of factors, such as:

► *Infection.*
► *Other glandular problems, particularly concerning the pituitary gland which controls the adrenal gland to a great extent.*
► *Addison's disease, or a direct failure of the adrenal glands.*
► *Tumours, especially in major organs or glands, leading to an alteration of the hormonal system.*

can cause a wide range of symptoms. Hypofunction symptoms include dehydration with a consequent drop in blood pressure and risk of shock, hypoglycaemia (see page 144–5), weakness, dizziness, weight loss and recurrent infections. Symptoms of excessive production include muscle wasting, weight gain and redistribution of fat to the trunk and upper back, menstrual problems, excessive facial hair, mental disorders and mood swings. Production of some adrenal hormones is also influenced by the pituitary gland. Because of this, a tumour or other pituitary disorder can also lead to excess or reduced production of adrenal hormones, requiring proper medical attention.

SYMPTOMS

► Dehydration
► Drop in blood pressure
► Tiredness and fatigue
► Difficulty concentrating and dizziness
► Muscle wasting
► Weight gain or loss
► Recurrent infections

DIETARY MANAGEMENT

The adrenal glands depend not only on good quality nutrients for their optimum function, but also healthy activity on the part of the other glands in the endocrine system, such as the thyroid and pituitary. All these glands are strengthened by following a diet that provides an abundance of dark green leafy vegetables, complex carbohydrates, and good protein from sources such as egg yolk and soya products.

Rather than trying to increase sodium by taking table salt (which can lead to excess sodium consumption and result in high blood pressure and water retention), include natural sodium-rich foods, such as celery, beetroot, strawberries, almonds and spinach in your diet.

The diet should also contain foods to support the bacteria of the gut which are responsible for producing vitamins such as pantothenic acid (vitamin B_5). Vegetable fibre provides a matrix for the acidophilus bacteria which colonise the gut, while they may be replenished by bacteria-rich lactic-fermented foods, such as miso, tofu, live yoghurt, and lacto-fermented juices. Celery juice is considered by some dietitians to be good for the adrenal glands. An alternative is to mix carrot juice with raw goat's milk and take a wineglassful three times a day before meals.

Have regular meals that are high in complex carbohydrates, and limit intake of sugar, tea, coffee and alcohol to prevent fluctuations in blood sugar levels and minimise the stress on the adrenals. Snacking in between meals can be a good way of balancing your energy levels. Try eating nuts and fruit when you feel your energy levels draining a few hours after a meal. This will also help you to keep going until your next meal.

SUPPLEMENTS

Supplements can help to ensure a proper intake of certain nutrients.

▶ *Several of the B vitamins, notably folic acid, B_5 and B_{12}, may protect against exhaustion.*

▶ *Vitamin C levels are significantly reduced under stressful conditions. Take 500 mg daily.*

▶ *Coenzyme Q10 as a supplement is thought to help various forms of fatigue and adrenal exhaustion, although there is no conclusive evidence. Take 30 mg daily.*

▶ *Magnesium plays an important role in regulating energy metabolism. Take 250 mg daily in the form of magnesium phosphate.*

▶ *Potassium is crucial for neuromuscular coordination, and additional quantities are needed in cases of fatigue. Use in a physiologically balanced formula combined with magnesium.*

HERBAL MEDICINE

Several herbs are reputed to assist the body's adaptation to stressful situations. Principal among these is ginseng (*Panax ginseng*), which contains a group of compounds known as adaptogens.

Adaptogens promote and support the body's adaptive mechanisms to stressful situations or extra physical demands. Ginseng is widely available and may be taken for periods of three to four weeks at a time, followed by a break of at least two weeks before

GINSENG
Care should be taken when using ginseng – if you take too much you can get an adrenaline rush or find it difficult to sleep at night.

commencing a course again. Other herbal extracts which support the adrenal glands include wild yam (*Dioscorea villosa*) and liquorice (*Glycyrrhiza glabra*).

Consult a medical herbalist for advice on the most appropriate combinations of these and other herbs for your individual needs.

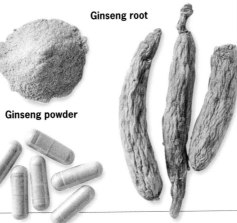

Ginseng root

Ginseng powder

Ginseng tablets

HOMEOPATHY

Homeopathy aims to cure an illness or condition through minute doses of plant extracts and other naturally occurring materials. The following remedies can help to treat adrenal deficiency and should be taken in low potencies for a few weeks. Check your symptoms for the right remedy, and see your doctor if symptoms persist. Calcaria carbonicum 6 should be taken if you have a sallow complexion, cold extremities, nausea, anorexia and insomnia. Natrum muriaticum 6 is for a yellow complexion, brown spots on the backs of the hands, lassitude, cold extremities and tension in the kidney region. Sepia 6 should be taken for weakness, fainting, yellow complexion, nausea at the smell of food, weak back and restless limbs.

Thyroid Problems

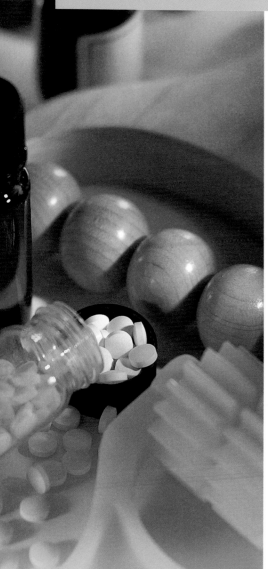

The thyroid gland is in direct control of your metabolic rate and energy levels. Thyroid disorders are often easily treated with orthodox medication. Complementary therapies and self-help measures can also help to relieve symptoms and boost health.

THE PROBLEMS

The thyroid gland is situated at the front of the neck, just below and in front of the voice box. It produces two hormones which regulate the rate at which the cells convert food into energy – triiodothyronine (T3) and thyroxin (T4). When the gland is underactive (hypothyroidism) it does not produce sufficient T3 or T4 and soon one or more symptoms may become evident. Because there are a number of possible causes for the symptoms of thyroid problems, the condition is often overlooked.

Overactivity of the thyroid gland (hyperthyroidism) results in excessive thyroxin which overstimulates body functions. Swelling of the thyroid gland (goitre) can occur in hyperthyroidism and hypothyroidism, but it is more common in the former.

Disturbance of the gland can have serious consequences for your health, so medical advice is essential, but some natural medicine measures can play an important supportive role in dealing with the condition.

Your doctor can arrange blood tests to check the levels of T4 and thyroid stimulating hormone (TSH). A deficiency of the free T4 (that which is available to the body), accompanied by an increase of TSH, indicates thyroid deficiency. If the figures for T4 are lower than an acceptable level, your doctor may need to prescribe thyroxin tablets. In borderline cases – such as those with normal test results but a persistence of symptoms – nutritional and herbal support may be effective.

If there are indications of an overactive thyroid, conventional treatment will be with drugs which suppress T4 or, in severe cases, surgical removal of part or all of the gland. When this is done thyroxin may need to be taken for life to make up for the created deficiency.

Regular medical monitoring and treatment of thyroid function is essential, but some symptoms can be helped by natural therapy measures with professional guidance.

THYROID FACTORS

For the thyroid gland to function properly it needs enzymes, protein and iodine, which are vital for the production of T3 and T4 hormones. Thyroid stimulating hormone (TSH) is produced by the pituitary gland, and pituitary problems can also cause thyroid disorders.

The thyroid can be adversely affected by antibodies produced by the immune system, known as an autoimmune disorder. In Hashimoto's thyroiditis, the antibodies destroy the thyroid gland, resulting in hypothyroidism. In Grave's disease, the antibodies stimulate the thyroid to produce excessive amounts of hormones, leading to hyperthyroidism.

SYMPTOMS

Of hypothyroidism:
- Lethargy and lack of energy
- Weight gain
- Dry skin, thinning hair and nails
- Voice changes
- Constipation
- Feelings of chilliness

Of hyperthyroidism:
- Palpitations and sweating
- Weight loss
- Staring or protruding eyes

DIETARY ADVICE

These guidelines can be applied for most cases of thyroid imbalance, but also consult a doctor or naturopath.

Add iodine
Although iodine is added to table salt, some diets can be deficient in this mineral. Sardines and other saltwater fish, seaweed, wheat germ, nuts, seeds and live goat's milk yoghurt are all rich sources of iodine and other nutrients.

Cut down on refined foods
Avoid refined foods, especially sugar, white flour and the de-natured grains. Imbalances of blood sugar levels affect metabolism greatly.

Limit stimulants
Limit consumption of coffee, strong tea, cola and alcohol, especially if you suffer from hyperthyroidism.

Eat fruit and vegetables
Fresh raw fruit and vegetables should be taken on a daily basis to provide antioxidants (especially vitamins A, C and E), and the nutrients needed for effective liver detoxification.

Consume vital fatty acids
Ensure that you eat regular food sources of the essential fatty acids from vegetable oils, tahini and sunflower or pumpkin seeds.

Aid the digestion
Live goat's or sheep's milk yoghurt or lacto-fermented vegetable juices need to be taken to top up the healthy bacteria in the gut. These promote nutrient assimilation and control food intolerance. Digestive disturbances, such as deficiency of enzymes, cause abdominal bloating and other intestinal disorders.

SUPPLEMENTS

Nutritional supplements of the more important antioxidant nutrients can help thyroid problems.

▶ *Vitamin B complex provides metabolic support for cases of hyperthyroidism, but may also be a general tonic for the tiredness of hypothyroidism. Use 100 mg daily of a good quality B complex.*

▶ *Up to 400 mg per day of magnesium orotate can help. Take as a combination with potassium.*

▶ *Vitamin E is an antioxidant and tonic to the circulation. Two capsules of 100 mg should be taken twice daily.*

▶ *Kelp is a herbal preparation of the seaweed* Fucus vesiculosus *('bladder rack'), which is a source of natural iodine.*

STRESS MANAGEMENT

The frequent pressures of emotional arousal and long-term stress or anxiety either overexcite an already excessively active thyroid, or place impossible demands on a deficient thyroid. It is worth taking steps to lower your level of arousal and help the nervous system to function at a less demanding pace.

This can be achieved partly by a healthy diet that excludes stimulants, such as coffee, strong tea and alcohol, but also by practising regular relaxation or meditation. Yoga classes may be a very good way of learning this as the gentle exercise and breathing routines of yoga are harmonising to body functions (see page 116). Bach flower remedies may also be of help (see page 46).

Aromatherapy massage, using essential oils, is also of value in the management of stress. A few drops of some oils can be added to a warm bath, or you can add a few drops to a teaspoonful of water in an oil burner.

*SELF-MASSAGE
The calming effects of massage with aromatherapy oils help to relieve stress.*

HOMEOPATHY
Homeopathy is a gentle and safe way of supporting conventional treatment for thyroid problems, but you must follow the instructions carefully. For individualised deeper-acting prescriptions, you should consult a homeopath, but the following remedies may help in appropriate circumstances:

▶ *Fucus 6 can help to bring T4 down. Take one tablet four times daily.*

▶ *Spongia 30 increases T4 and is good for treating swollen glands and hard phlegm in the throat and voice changes. Take one tablet twice daily.*

▶ *Iodum 30 raises T4 and can help an over-active thyroid and restlessness. Take one tablet twice daily for two weeks.*

▶ *Belladonna 6 also raises T4 and helps hot, flushed hyperthyroid sufferers. Take one tablet four times daily for four or five days.*

Diabetes

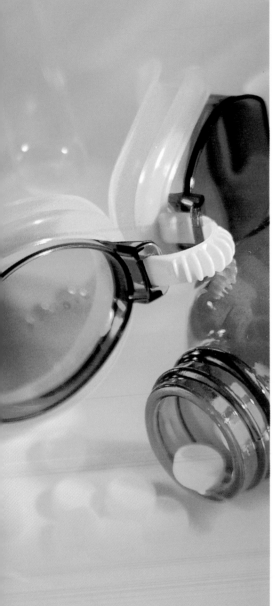

Diabetes can come on gradually, rendering the sufferer progressively more tired and less able to transform food into energy. Dietary measures can help to alleviate the problem, enabling you to resume a normal, healthy lifestyle.

THE PROBLEM

Insulin, produced in the pancreas, promotes the uptake of glucose into cells so that it can be metabolised to produce energy. When the process is disturbed, usually due to a lack of insulin, the blood sugar rises because it cannot get into the cells, resulting in diabetes.

There are two main types of diabetes. The severest form, called insulin-dependent, or type I, diabetes most often occurs in people under the age of 16. This type of diabetes needs to be treated with insulin injections and a strict diet.

The more common form, called non-insulin-dependent, or type II, diabetes generally occurs later in life, usually after the age of 40. It is relatively common, and often discovered only as a result of routine medical tests. It is thought that many people are suffering from a mild form of diabetes without realising it, with only one third of sufferers developing any symptoms. It is often treated by dietary measures alone.

Diet is the most important factor in the management of diabetes. After a meal the blood glucose level rises and insulin is needed to transport it into the body cells to be converted into energy. If the glucose cannot be transformed, the blood sugar rises to dangerous levels and the body cells are deprived of energy. Excess sugar is excreted in the urine where it can be detected by tests.

CAUSES OF DIABETES

Insulin-dependent diabetes is caused by the destruction of insulin-secreting cells in the pancreas. It tends to run in families and is thought to be caused by the immune system attacking the body's own tissues, possibly following a viral infection. It occurs most often in people under the age of 16.

Non-insulin-dependent diabetes is caused by a reduction in the amount of insulin that is produced by the body, or because the body has become resistant to its effects. It is more common in overweight people, and those over the age of 40.

It is important that diabetics follow a strict dietary regime in order to balance carbohydrate consumption with insulin intake. The aim is to avoid sudden swings in blood sugar levels. This often requires discipline that can be hard to maintain, especially in children. In particular, diabetics should limit their intake of simple sugars which pass rapidly into the bloodstream and cause a sudden rise in blood glucose levels. It is important to eat breakfast, lunch and an evening meal. Those taking insulin or tablets may need snacks between meals and before bed. Your dietitian will provide dietary guidelines on the right amount of carbohydrate to eat at each meal.

SYMPTOMS

▶ Tiredness and possibly dizziness and fainting

▶ Unusual thirst

▶ Excessive urination

▶ Weight loss

▶ Poor resistance to infections

▶ Tingling in the hands and feet

▶ Deterioration of eyesight

DIETARY MEASURES FOR DIABETICS

A number of measures are used to help to control blood glucose levels.

Reduce sugar

Simple sugars (glucose and sucrose) and foods which contain them, such as chocolates and fruit drinks, should be consumed sparingly and, when possible, in combination with a complex carbohydrate.

Carbohydrates

Obtain your main sources of energy from complex carbohydrates, such as bread, potatoes and rice. Products such as buckwheat, millet, brown rice and rye bread are high in fibre and so are absorbed more steadily by the digestive system.

Fruit and vegetables

Fresh fruit and vegetables are important sources of vitamins, minerals and fibre. Eat at least five portions every day.

Protein sources

Protein from plant sources such as legumes, especially soya products, provide additional fibre and should be included in the diet together with moderate animal protein intake from lean meats, fish and dairy produce.

Limit fat levels

Restrict fat to 15–20 per cent of the diet, and obtain it mainly from plant sources such as seeds, nuts and polyunsaturated vegetable oils.

HERBAL TREATMENT

A number of medicinal plants promote or support the functions of organs and tissues at risk from diabetes, while there are also several which have an antidiabetic action.

The heart and circulation can be sustained with the help of hawthorn berries (*Crataegus oxyacantha*) and gingko biloba, which is reputed to be protective against diabetic retinopathy – a disease affecting the retinas. The liver can be helped by using barberry (*Berberis vulgaris*), the digestive system can be improved by using ginger (*Zingiber officinalis*) and wild

*ANTIDIABETIC HERBS
Plants reputed to have this property include garlic (*Allium cepa) and stinging nettle (*Urtica dioica). Careful regulation is essential to maintain adequate blood sugar levels, especially if you are taking drugs or insulin for your diabetes.*

yam (*Dioscorea villosa*), and the nervous system may be regulated with skullcap (*Scutellaria laterifolia*) and valerian (*Valeriana officinalis*).

Antidiabetic herbs can help to reduce blood sugar levels and free up spare insulin.

SUPPLEMENTS

Recent research in nutritional biochemistry has emphasised the importance of specific nutrients in stabilising blood sugar levels, as well as helping to protect tissues susceptible to damage in diabetics. The heart and blood vessels and nervous system, and the retinas in the eyes, are particularly vulnerable in diabetics and antioxidant nutrients can help to prevent their deterioration. It may be worth consulting a naturopath or a doctor who practises nutritional medicine for individual prescriptions and recommendations, especially if you are an insulin-dependent diabetic.

▶ *Chromium combines with other nutrients to form what is known as the glucose tolerance factor, which is particularly important for elderly diabetics. Glucose tolerance factor is found in brewer's yeast and you may need to take up to 20 brewer's yeast tablets every day to satisfy your body's needs.*

▶ *Vitamin C is necessary for healthy tissues, especially those of the blood vessels, and to regulate cholesterol levels which are inclined to be higher in diabetics. Take 500 to 1000 mg daily, preferably in two doses, one with breakfast in the morning and the other with your evening meal, in the form of bioflavonoid complex.*

▶ *Multimineral supplements containing plenty of magnesium, potassium and zinc – all of which are important to regulate blood sugar levels – should be taken daily. Practitioners may recommend additional supplements with individual minerals and trace elements.*

▶ *Evening primrose oil can help with metabolising essential fatty acids and boosting energy levels. This can be very useful since many diabetics tend to be less efficient at this process.*

Hypoglycaemia

Hypoglycaemia occurs when there is a low blood sugar level, causing persistent tiredness. Dietary control is one of the primary methods of countering the condition, ensuring that your sugar and carbohydrate intakes remain balanced.

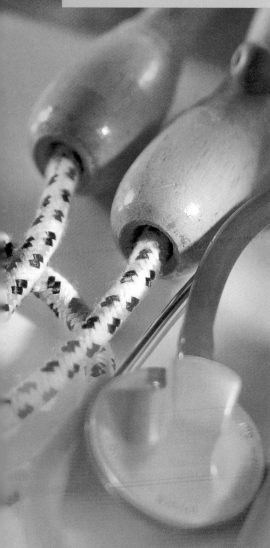

THE PROBLEM

The brain and other tissues of the body require a steady supply of glucose for energy. This is derived from food, but in order for it to be taken up by the cells insulin, a hormone secreted by the pancreas, is necessary. A lack of insulin causes hyperglycaemia (excess sugar in the blood) which is a sign of diabetes (see page 142). If too much insulin is produced, the blood sugar level falls and the brain and body are deprived of energy, leading to hypoglycaemia. This is less critical for the muscles and body tissues than it is for the brain, which requires the greater part of our energy output.

Constant overproduction of insulin through excessive intake of sugary foods, which is known as hyperinsulinism, can cause the body tissues to become gradually more resistant to its influence. The wide range of symptoms thought to be due to insulin resistance have become known as syndrome X. They include chronic fatigue, allergies, headaches, migraines, loss of concentration and irritability, as well as heart disease and high blood pressure.

The most accurate way of diagnosing hypoglycaemia is by a five-hour glucose tolerance test which measures the blood sugar levels at regular intervals up to five hours after taking a concentrated glucose solution. When positive, the blood sugar level actually falls below

HYPOGLYCAEMIA FACTORS

There are three main types of hypoglycaemia, probably the most common being experienced by diabetics who fail to eat regularly and experience a rapid fall of blood sugar levels. Reactive hypoglycaemia occurs when a fall in blood sugar levels is caused by foods which induce an oversecretion of insulin by the pancreas. The third main type of hypoglycaemia are tumours of the pancreas or pituitary gland which can alter insulin levels, causing a fall in blood sugar levels.

Hypoglycaemia often follows periods of high physical or emotional demand. The chances of hypoglycaemia can be increased by the overconsumption of refined foods, caffeine, alcohol and sugar which produce a roller coaster rise and fall of blood sugar levels.

the fasting level after about two-and-a-half to three hours and may be accompanied by headaches or feelings of faintness. The rate of fall of the blood sugar level and the recovery, as compensatory mechanisms take over, give the practitioner important information about the type of hypoglycaemia.

It is also possible to diagnose hypoglycaemia on the basis of clinical signs and symptoms.

SYMPTOMS

▶ Dizziness and fainting
▶ Lack of concentration
▶ Headaches or migraines, especially on rising
▶ Palpitations
▶ Irritability and mood swings
▶ Depression
▶ Persistent tiredness
▶ Susceptibility to allergies and intolerances
▶ Cravings for sweets, cigarettes and alcohol

DIETARY MANAGEMENT

An important way of regulating hypoglycaemia is to control excess insulin production and this can only be achieved through dietary modification. For proper diagnosis of low blood sugar and dietary management, consult a doctor specialising in nutritional medicine or a naturopath. The following guidelines can be helpful at home.

Avoid refined foods

Avoid foods which release sugar too rapidly and overstimulate the pancreas – including all refined carbohydrates, especially sugar and white flour. Also avoid stimulants, particularly products that contain caffeine, such as coffee, tea and soft drinks. The imbalancing effects of alcohol can influence your hormone production, and tobacco may also have an overstimulating effect.

Complex carbohydrates

Eat foods that are absorbed slowly and can sustain energy levels, such as a high-fibre or high-complex carbohydrate diet.

Do not miss meals

Eat smaller meals and have a high-carbohydrate snack between the main meals at mid morning, mid afternoon and last thing at night. This can help to avoid energy swings before and after meals.

Lifestyle and metabolism

Take regular physical exercise, building up the amount gradually. Also practise a good relaxation routine, and learn to take deep breaths – a tendency to hyperventilate, taking rapid shallow breaths, is common among hypoglycaemic people.

Nutritional supplements are no substitute for a healthy diet, but when used in conjunction with a balanced range of foods they can help to avoid fluctuations in blood sugar levels. Vitamin B, magnesium, potassium, manganese, chromium and zinc all play major roles in blood sugar regulation.

If you have pronounced symptoms of hypoglycaemia, you should consult a practitioner and have the appropriate tests. The commonly used tests for trace elements and minerals in blood serum are not such reliable indicators of their availability to the body as testing the sweat or red blood cells.

The following supplements may be needed for hypoglycaemia regulation and may be taken for three to six months at a time. Longer term supplementation may be required by chronic sufferers of the syndrome.

▶ *Vitamin B complex at a dosage of 100 mg per day.*

▶ *A 500 mg tablet of vitamin C can be taken 3 or 4 times daily.*

▶ *Magnesium doses of 200–400 mg per day, as magnesium orotate or physiologically balanced magnesium phosphate.*

▶ *Potassium, 500 mg per day, as a combination or as potassium phosphate, the physiologically balanced form.*

▶ *Take 25 mg of zinc at night before going to bed.*

▶ *Chromium is one of the most important nutrients and combines with other compounds to form the glucose tolerance factor that is found in brewer's yeast. Brewer's yeast tablets supply the necessary factor, or preparations of chromium with magnesium and potassium can be taken. The recommended dose is 200 µg every day.*

ENERGY-BOOSTING SNACKS

Snacking between meals ensures that you keep your blood sugar levels balanced. While it is often easier to reach for a chocolate bar or piece of cake, your snacks should be more nutritious. Foods high in complex carbohydrates, particularly grains, are dissolved slowly, giving you a constant stream of fuel to carry you through to the next meal. The best high-energy snacks include: fruit, nuts and seeds, dried fruit, chopped raw vegetables (carrots, baby corn, peppers, cauliflower, celery) either on their own or with dips, rice cakes, wholemeal crackers or bread, low-calorie wholemeal breakfast cereals, low-fat yoghurts, a small piece of cheese, a portion of cottage cheese, or a wholemeal bread roll with a low-fat filling.

ENERGY FOODS
You can eat as many pieces of fresh fruit and vegetables as you like to keep your energy levels high.

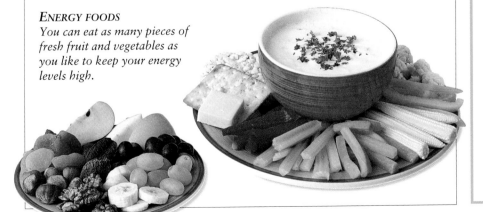

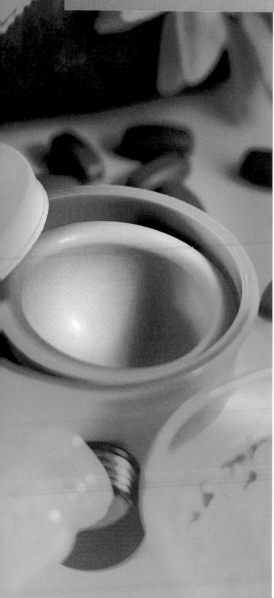

Cancer

Cancer is now the main overall cause of death in the UK and Western Europe, and it can affect people of all ages – although it is more common in older age groups. Understanding the many possible causes of cancer can help you to take steps to avoid it.

THE PROBLEM

Cancer is an uncontrolled growth of cells, or tumour, in a part of the body. It most often affects the lungs, breasts, skin, reproductive organs, stomach, large bowel, pancreas and the blood and bone marrow (leukaemia). The tumour grows and spreads into the surrounding tissues, where it destroys nerves and erodes bones. It may also travel to other parts of the body through the blood vessels or lymphatic system to set up metastases, or satellite tumours.

The hallmark of a cancerous or 'malign' tumour is that it spreads. A tumour that does not spread is said to be 'benign' and considered to be less dangerous, although it may still be life threatening if it presses on a vital organ such as the brain. Early symptoms of cancer vary enormously according to the site of the tumour. General fatigue and unexplained weight loss are common symptoms of the early stages of many types of cancer. Pain is often not an early symptom, although it should always be investigated by your doctor.

The main trigger factors are alcohol, smoking, sunlight, diet – especially ones high in animal fats or smoked products – and pollutants found in the environment that are breathed in or consumed in food and drinking water. Some people are at particular risk for genetic reasons.

Many cancers that occur in adulthood are also related to changes in the cells due to natural ageing. Young people, under 20 years old, are the least likely to contract cancer; the probability doubles after 30 and increases steadily throughout life. By the time a person reaches 90, there is a strong likelihood that he or she will have developed some form of cancer, although it may remain dormant and without symptoms.

Cancer is now the most common cause of death in the UK, accounting for one-fifth of all deaths. It has been identified since ancient times and also occurs throughout the animal kingdom.

Orthodox treatment for cancer can include one or more of the following: powerful drugs (chemotherapy), radiation (radiotherapy) and surgery. Many people include complementary health therapies to help to boost the immune system and to alleviate some of the symptoms of cancer as well as the side effects of treatment.

Some of the most effective complementary therapies are thought to be homeopathy and herbal treatments. A healthy and nutritious diet that includes plenty of antioxidant vitamins, found in fresh fruit and vegetables and wholegrain cereals, will also strengthen the body. Visualisation and art therapy, which are designed to focus the individual's own mental and physical resources on destroying the cancer, have also shown remarkable results.

SYMPTOMS

Cancer can cause a wide range of possible symptoms, including:

► Fatigue and rapid weight loss
► A persistent sore or ulcer
► A mole that changes size
► Severe headaches or persistent abdominal pain
► Blood in urine
► Changes to, or unexplained lumps in, the breasts or testicles
► Vaginal bleeding or spotting

FACTORS INFLUENCING THE RISK OF CANCER

Food and diet
Up to 70 per cent of cancers are thought to be linked to diet. In particular, a diet that is high in animal fats and refined sugar increases the risk of breast cancer. Stomach cancer is highest in countries like Japan where a lot of smoked foods are eaten. Bowel cancer is most common in countries such as the US with low-fibre diets.

Environment
The most common environmental cause of cancer is ultraviolet light from the sun. This can cause skin cancers such as malignant melanoma. Less common factors include asbestos, and radioactivity – both natural and man-made.

Smoking and alcohol
Smoking is by far the most common cause of lung cancer. Excess alcohol consumption increases the risk of cancers of the oesophagus (gullet), stomach and liver.

Genetic
Some genes, passed on from one generation to the next, make it more likely that certain tissues, especially in the female reproductive organs, may turn cancerous. So far only a few 'cancer genes' have been found, representing a minority of cancers.

Viral
The human papilloma virus, which causes genital warts, has been strongly linked to cervical cancer, and the hepatitis B virus can cause liver cancer. Infection by the human immunodeficiency virus (HIV) increases the risk of developing a range of cancers. Other viruses may also cause cancer but in many cases the link is not clear. These viruses are most commonly contracted through unprotected sexual intercourse.

A HEALTHY DIET

The main secret of a healthy diet is balance and moderation. Avoid excessive consumption of animal fats, such as meat and dairy foods, refined sugars and smoked meat, fish and cheese. Also avoid highly processed foods and those with large quantities of additives. Eat plenty of different kinds of fruit and vegetables to ensure the maximum intake of anticancer vitamins, or antioxidants. Eat plenty of high-fibre foods, such as pulses and wholegrain cereals. Fibre speeds waste products through the digestive tract and reduces the time that cancer-causing substances are in contact with the body. A diet that is high in soya products, such as soya beans and tofu, is thought to reduce the risk of breast cancer, although this is not proved.

PREVENTION OF SKIN CANCER

Skin cancer affects a large number of people every year, especially those with fair skin who have not protected themselves against the harmful ultraviolet rays of the sun. Staying out of the sun, wearing protective clothes or using sun block cream can all prevent skin cancer forming in this way. Cancerous spots, moles and warts can be easily treated if you spot their growth early.

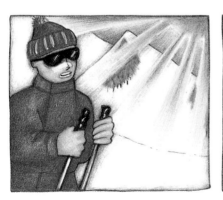

A holiday in the snow can be surprisingly dangerous for skin cancer. This is because the snow reflects the sun's rays, increasing the amount of ultraviolet rays.

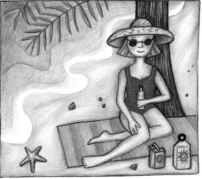

A holiday in the sun can be highly dangerous for fair-skinned people, particularly those with very pale skin that burns easily. Sunbathe carefully with good protection.

LIFESTYLE FACTORS

The best way to reduce the risk of contracting cancer is to follow a healthy lifestyle. This means both ensuring that the body is as fit as possible and also avoiding those factors known to increase the cancer risk. Regular moderate exercise, such as frequent brisk walks of at least 20 minutes' duration, will strengthen the body's immune system – but make sure exercise does not become excessive, which has the opposite effect on your health. Avoid smoking and keep alcohol consumption at moderate levels.

Women should examine their breasts regularly, and men should examine their testicles, to check for lumps or other abnormalities. Women should also have regular cervical smear tests.

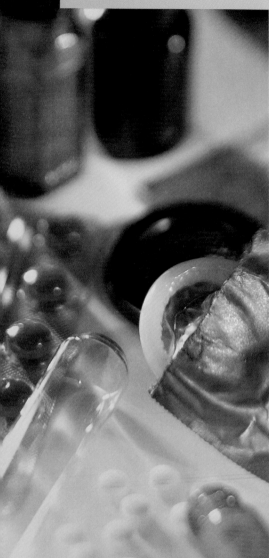

HIV and AIDS

AIDS is an incurable disorder that is caused by the HIV virus. Certain groups in society are particularly vulnerable to the condition, but everyone is at potential risk and must take proper precautions to avoid infection and the spread of the virus.

THE PROBLEM

AIDS stands for acquired immune deficiency syndrome. As the word syndrome indicates, it covers a wide range of possible disorders which may be contracted following the breakdown of the immune system. AIDS is caused by infection by the human immunodeficiency virus (HIV), which is most commonly contracted through infected blood, semen, or vaginal secretions. More rarely it may be passed on from mother to baby during childbirth or breastfeeding, although this can usually be avoided. In the past, HIV has also been contracted from infected blood and blood products used in medicine. This is no longer a risk as blood donors are screened and blood products are heat-treated to kill the virus.

AIDS first came to the attention of doctors in 1981, when a rare lung infection affecting previously healthy homosexual men in the US was reported. A series of infections, mostly rare in people with properly functioning immune systems, spread throughout this small community, and were also found in intravenous drug users and haemophiliacs, suggesting that infection was via the blood. In 1984, US and French researchers identified the virus, which became known as HIV.

HIV targets white cells called T4 cells found in the bloodstream which are a vital line of defence against

CAUSES OF INFECTION

The virus can be passed from person to person through a variety of ways, including:

► *Unprotected sexual intercourse with an infected person.*

► *Blood transfusion with infected blood (now very rare).*

► *Through the uterus, blood or breast milk of an infected mother.*

► *Using contaminated intravenous needles.*

disease. The immune system is seriously weakened, leaving the sufferer highly vulnerable to a range of opportunistic infections and cancers that a healthy person would probably fight off. HIV may also damage the brain and nervous system directly.

The interval between contracting HIV and developing the syndrome in its most serious form, known as 'full-blown AIDS', can be months or even years. Some people may develop a milder condition called AIDS-related complex (ARC) when they may have periods of good health interspersed with periods of illness. Many people with HIV infection do not show symptoms and yet will be infectious. This emphasises the need to stop the spread of the disease by following precautions which can easily be understood and adopted.

SYMPTOMS

Leading minor symptoms include:

► Skin disorders

► Unexplained weight loss

► Diarrhoea

► Fever

Severe symptoms include a susceptibility to infections, such as:

► Herpes

► Shingles

► Tuberculosis

► Cancerous tumours

DIAGNOSING AND TREATING HIV AND AIDS

HIV infection is diagnosed by means of a blood test to detect antibodies – antigerm chemicals – that the body produces to fight the disease. Those with HIV antibodies are said to be HIV-positive. There is no absolute cure and so HIV-positive people are infected for life and will always be able to pass it on. The test may give a false negative if done within two to three months of infection, before antibodies have developed, or late in the disease, when the immune system has broken down completely.

Orthodox treatment for HIV infection and AIDS includes antiviral drugs such as acyclovir and zidovudine (AZT). Other drugs and treatments may be given to treat specific symptoms. Current medical treatments can extend the life of sufferers by several years, many more in a number of cases, and new methods and treatments are being

discovered all the time which are further improving the outlook for sufferers and their families.

Complementary health systems can also provide useful additional care. In particular they can help to strengthen the immune system and alleviate some of the symptoms. They include herbal and traditional Chinese medicine, and homeopathic treatment. It is important to seek advice from a qualified practitioner and not attempt self-treatment.

In addition, sufferers should boost their own health and strengthen their immune system by following a healthy lifestyle. For example, take regular moderate exercise, and manage your stress levels, which can further impair your immune system. Eat a healthy, nutritious diet that is low in animal fats, sugar and refined foods and high in wholegrain cereals and rice, fresh fruit and vegetables.

HAVING A TEST

Should I have an HIV test?
It is very important to have a test for HIV if you think there is a chance that you may have become infected, or you are in a high-risk group. These include homosexuals and intravenous drug users. If you are thinking of having a test, seek counselling first to help you to comprehend the implications of a positive test result.

Where do I get an HIV test?
Your own doctor can carry out a blood test for HIV. However, if you prefer, tests for HIV are available at genitourinary medicine (GUM) clinics. The test result is totally confidential and the doctor or the clinic staff can give you counselling as well as medical advice and treatment.

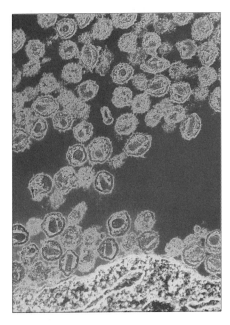

HIV VIRUS
The HIV virus affects the white blood cells, gradually crippling the immune system and leaving weak points that allow infections to take hold. The more common infections that can easily breach a weakened immune system include herpes, shingles and tuberculosis.

AVOIDING HIV INFECTION

The most important defence against contracting HIV is the practice of safe sex. This is particularly important for people with several sexual partners or if you are starting a new relationship with someone who has had other sexual partners. The greatest risk is from having penetrative anal or vaginal sex, so it follows that by only practising sexual activities such as oral sex, mutual masturbation, hugging, stroking or petting you are significantly reducing the chances of infection. If you have a friend who is HIV positive, do remember that you cannot be infected by hugging or touching.

When having penetrative sex, it is advisable to use a condom to act as a barrier to vaginal and seminal secretions. These precautions against infection are not necessary in well-established, mutually monogamous relationships.

Intravenous drug users should avoid sharing needles, syringes or other injection equipment. In areas of Britain with a high rate of intravenous drug use, needles and syringes are often provided free by local health centres in order to prevent the spread of HIV.

High-risk activities include:
▶ *Sharing needles and syringes with an intravenous drug user.*
▶ *Having unprotected sex with someone whose sexual history is unknown to you.*

Low or no-risk activities include:
▶ *Penetrative sex within a mutually monogamous relationship.*
▶ *Non-penetrative sex.*
▶ *Using public toilets.*
▶ *Donating blood.*
▶ *Kissing an infected person.*
▶ *Sharing plates or eating utensils with an infected person.*

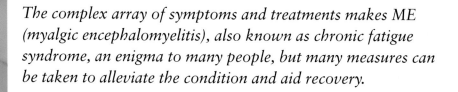

ME (Chronic Fatigue Syndrome)

The complex array of symptoms and treatments makes ME (myalgic encephalomyelitis), also known as chronic fatigue syndrome, an enigma to many people, but many measures can be taken to alleviate the condition and aid recovery.

THE PROBLEM

ME, also known as chronic fatigue syndrome (CFS), is a complex illness mainly involving the muscles and nervous system. A major feature of the condition is muscular aching and an inability to concentrate. The onset of the symptoms often follows a viral illness, so another name in common use is post-viral fatigue syndrome.

In the US, the disorder is referred to by the more comprehensive term chronic fatigue immune deficiency syndrome (CFIDS) or chronic Epstein-Barr virus (EBV), named after the disease responsible for one of the major viral illnesses, glandular fever, which frequently precedes the syndrome. In the UK, the Royal College of Physicians has formally adopted the term chronic fatigue syndrome.

The collection of names simply emphasises how imprecise a condition it is; the symptoms affect the whole body, but because no single pathological cause can be found to account for it, CFS is regarded as a controversial illness. Sufferers are often described as depressive and the disorder is often labelled as psychosomatic. Many ME patients are often depressed, but this is usually a symptom of fatigue and not the underlying cause.

Just as the diagnosis of ME is controversial so, too, is its treatment. No single therapy or system of medicine can be said to have a satisfactory solution to the problem, although many treatments can be helpful when used as part of an integrated approach. Diet and nutrition are among the more popular and successful ways of dealing with ME and some of the side effects associated with fatigue. Other complementary therapies, such as homeopathy and herbal remedies, are also used to help to moderate some of the symptoms. Rest and relaxation exercises have been known to play a significant role in some cases of recovery, and many sufferers have found their own personal relaxation remedies.

CAUSES OF ME

There is no single cause of ME, but a number of factors which undermine the immunity and energy metabolism may combine to precipitate the illness. Among these are the following:

▶ *Recurrent viral illnesses or periods of stress.*
▶ *Insufficient sleep.*
▶ *Poor nutrition.*
▶ *Weakness of digestive functions.*
▶ *Hypoglycaemia.*
▶ *Intestinal candidiasis (yeast overgrowth).*
▶ *Impaired liver function.*
▶ *Leaky gut.*

SYMPTOMS

ME can be responsible for a combination of the following symptoms:

▶ Tiredness and lack of concentration
▶ Muscle aches and pains
▶ Recurrent infections
▶ Headaches
▶ Insomnia
▶ Increased sensitivity to light and sound

MANAGEMENT OF ME

Because of the need to focus on the underlying problems in a direct way, ME sufferers should always seek professional advice. ME is a syndrome – a collection of symptoms – and there is no definitive test for it, but a number of functional disorders may account for many of its symptoms and can be investigated using tests which are not usually carried out in conventional medical diagnosis. Among these may be tests for adrenal insufficiency, hypothyroidism, hypoglycaemia, disorders of liver function, deficiencies of digestive enzymes, intestinal candidiasis, and vitamin and mineral deficiencies. One or more of these disorders are commonly present in the ME patient.

Chronic fatigue is the consequence of a number of possible ways in which energy production and nerve function has become obstructed or impaired by viral infection or damage to the immune system. The sequence of physiological and biochemical reactions requires specific nutrients at various stages.

Nutrition

Dietary advice and nutritional supplements are often important components of ME management. A person with ME needs a diet that meets a number of criteria – but a balanced food intake is of little value if the means of digesting and absorbing it are impaired. It would, therefore, be advisable to consult a nutritionally trained doctor or a naturopath who can arrange for appropriate treatment. Advice can then be given on the most suitable dietary measures.

Most nutrients are provided by a balanced, wholefood diet, but when the need for specific factors is greater, or where digestive efficiency is poor, supplements may be helpful. Patients with ME can be persuaded of the need for almost every imaginable nutrient and hefty programmes of supplements are of little value if the means to digest and assimilate them are impaired. The best plan is to seek professional advice so that nutritional needs can be identified on the basis of proper investigation.

Herbal medicines can give valuable support for a number of aspects of the problem.

Exercise

According to some authorities, excessive aerobic exercise will worsen the condition of the ME patient. Dr Paul Cheney, a leading authority in the US, says patients with this disease cannot be trained aerobically unless they are well on the way to recovery. Aerobic exercise, such as running, swimming and cycling, must therefore be strictly rationed. Some studies suggest that graded daily exercise, such as walking or gentle swimming, building up the amount by small weekly increments, can help. Anaerobic exercise such as weightlifting seems to be more manageable for short periods.

UNSTRENUOUS EXERCISE
Singing is great for your lungs and improves your heartbeat, your blood oxygen levels and your sense of well-being, without being too exhausting. If you find it too tiring to stand up, you can always sit down while you sing, provided you keep your back straight. Joining an amateur choir or singing group is both good exercise for your cardiovascular system and an excellent way to reduce stress.

DIETARY TIPS

The following dietary tips have proved beneficial in many cases of ME. However, always consult your doctor or a qualified nutritionist before making major changes in your diet.

▶ *Use unrefined complex carbohydrates such as wholemeal flour, brown rice, millet, couscous and quinoa.*

▶ *Have a mixed raw salad as one of your daily meals.*

▶ *Operate the five-a-day rule – eat at least five servings of raw fruit or vegetables every day.*

▶ *Vary your protein intake with more pulses, nuts, seeds and tofu, in place of meat, eggs and cheese. If you are not vegetarian, oily fish once a week is permissible.*

▶ *Aim for smaller, more frequent meals rather than overeating at main meals. Carry some sunflower or pumpkin seeds as a top-up snack in case you have to miss or delay a meal.*

▶ *Avoid caffeine, alcohol and grapefruit which overactivate the first phase of liver detoxification, producing more potent toxic compounds.*

▶ *Avoid sugar and foods which contain it, such as cakes, sweets, biscuits and chocolate, which are a potential challenge to the digestive system.*

A MENU FOR ME

This menu planner will give you some idea of the variety of foods which will provide a range of essential nutrients, while avoiding foods that place stress on the liver, pancreas and intestines. If you have intolerances to any food, be sure to avoid it. If you think you might have an allergy to a certain food, keep a diary of how you feel when you have eaten it; if you notice any ill effects, cut it out of your diet. By monitoring the effects of different foods, you can work out those which are best for you.

On rising
► Cup of hot water with a dessertspoonful of apple cider vinegar or a teaspoonful of fresh lemon juice and half a teaspoonful of honey; or one tisane of peppermint tea.

Breakfast
► A herb tea such as peppermint or lemon and ginger, or a coffee substitute.

► Fresh fruit juice or a small glass of lactic-fermented juice.

► Home-made muesli, made by soaking organic porridge oats in a cup of water overnight. Add grated apple, sliced pear, raisins or sultanas, pumpkin or sunflower seeds and a dessertspoonful of light tahini.

► Live goat's or sheep's milk yoghurt.

Mid morning
► Cup of peppermint, camomile or rosehip tea.

► A double handful of sunflower seeds or a few brazil nuts or almonds. Alternatively, a rice cake with some cottage cheese or ricotta.

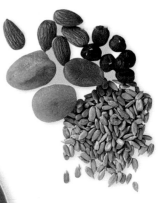

Lunch
► A mixed raw salad containing a selection of lettuce, watercress, parsley, white cabbage, chicory, cucumber, tomatoes and carrots. Add a dessertspoonful of ricotta or cottage cheese or a savoury nut slice. Garnish with pine kernels, raisins, or pumpkin seeds, and a dressing of extra virgin olive oil, cider vinegar, tahini and yoghurt.

► Rye biscuits, rice cakes, or wholemeal bread and a savoury spread, such as miso, or a baked potato with low-fat spread or hummous.

► Fresh fruit for dessert.

Dinner
► Aperitif of lactic-fermented beetroot or celery juice.

► A raw food appetiser of grated apple and carrot dressed with virgin olive oil and lemon juice; or crudités of carrot, pepper, celery, cauliflower or broccoli and a tofu or hummous dip.

► Main dish of fish, lean meat or a vegetarian option served with two or three steamed vegetables; or mixed vegetable stew with fresh ingredients; or a brown rice or wholemeal pasta dish. Do not fry the ingredients.

► Dessert of fresh fruit or soya-based dessert, soaked dried fruit, or jelly made with a seaweed base.

Mid afternoon
► A cup of herb tea or, if you prefer, a glass of fresh fruit juice.

► Seeds or nuts as a snack.

► A portion of fresh fruit, or a bowl of fresh fruit salad.

HERBAL TREATMENTS

A medical herbalist can select combinations of plant extracts according to the specific needs of the patient. Detoxification functions may be assisted by the use of barberry (*Berberis vulgaris*), pokeroot (*Phytolacca decandra*), especially for fatigue following glandular fever, and burdock (*Arctium lappa*). Barberry is also an organ remedy for the liver, while pokeroot improves lymphatic functions.

Irritated or weakened intestinal linings may impair absorption of nutrients and cause food intolerances. They can be assisted by extracts of liquorice (*Glycyrrhiza glabra*), which also supports the adrenal glands, marshmallow (*Althea officinalis*) and wild yam (*Dioscoroea villosa*). Among general tonics are kola (*Cola vera*), especially for muscle weakness, damiana (*Turnera diffusa*), also a useful aphrodisiac, and wild oats (*Avena sativa*). Ginger (*Zingiber officinalis*) may be used to assist the actions of the other herbs and is a good digestive tonic.

There are several herbs which may be tried without professional guidance including ginseng (*Panax ginseng*), gingko (*Gingko biloba*), which helps to improve circulation to the extremities, and coneflower (*Echinacea angustifolia*), which stimulates non-specific immunity. Any of these may be taken for two to three weeks at a time, followed by two to three weeks' break.

GLANDULAR FEVER

Glandular fever, which is also known as infectious mononucleosis, is commonly called the 'kissing disease' because it is often transmitted in the saliva through kissing. It is common among young people aged between 10 and 25 and so is more widespread among closed communities of young people, such as schools, colleges and universities. It causes severe fatigue, as well as fever, sore throat, swollen lymph nodes, general muscular aches and pains and depression. Orthodox treatment involves complete rest and regular consumption of warm drinks. Although it is usually contracted in early age, the Epstein-Barr virus (EBV) that causes the disease may stay in the body and cause recurrent bouts of fatigue, depression and illness throughout a person's life. Recognising the symptoms and taking it easy are two of the keys to management.

Dietary measures
Foods rich in vitamins and minerals that help to boost the immune system will hasten recovery. Vitamins include vitamin C found in fruit and vegetables; vitamin A found in liver, eggs, fish oils and low-fat dairy products; vitamin E found in wheatgerm, nuts, seeds and vegetable oils; and vitamin B complex found in lean meat, fish, soya, pulses, peanuts and wholegrain products. Minerals include copper, iron, selenium and zinc found in lean meat, fish, wholegrains, and brown rice. Some people may choose to take supplements, although care must be taken to ensure that overdoses are not reached. It is always better to eat a balanced diet to obtain all the nutrients you need naturally.

Homeopathy
A qualified homeopath will tailor the choice of remedy to the individual case. However, the following have proved effective in many cases: Ailanthus for rash and inflammation; Mercurious solubilis for swollen lymph nodes and fatigue; and Phytolacca for general aches and pains.

SUPPLEMENTS

You should seek a nutritionist's advice on your specific needs and which supplements would help to improve both your energy levels and the underlying condition. However, the following supplements will invariably be helpful in most cases of chronic fatigue:

▶ *Vitamin B complex, a yeast-free type, at a dose of 100 mg per day.*

▶ *Vitamin C taken at 500–1000 mg per day.*

▶ *Vitamin E can be taken as two capsules of an emulsified form of the 100 mg strength, taken twice daily.*

▶ *Magnesium is one of the most important nutrients for chronic fatigue. This should be taken as magnesium citrate, 200 mg daily, or the physiologically balanced form as magnesium phosphate combined with potassium phosphate, another important nutrient.*

▶ *Zinc may be taken as zinc citrate 50 mg, two tablets daily. Take zinc supplements at night, separately from other nutrients.*

▶ *Selenium is found in brewer's yeast, together with the glucose tolerance factor, chromium. Use brewer's yeast tablets if you do not have yeast-related digestive problems (candidiasis), otherwise use the commercially available combination of selenium with vitamins A and C. Selenium works closely with vitamin E, with which it should always be taken.*

▶ *Coenzyme Q10 may help, although there is no conclusive evidence to its beneficial qualities. A trial in Charing Cross Hospital found that Q10 supplements gave no definite benefit to ME sufferers. It may be helpful as a supplement in ME cases with muscle fatigue as a prominent feature. Recommended dose is 20–50 mg per day.*

Viral Infections

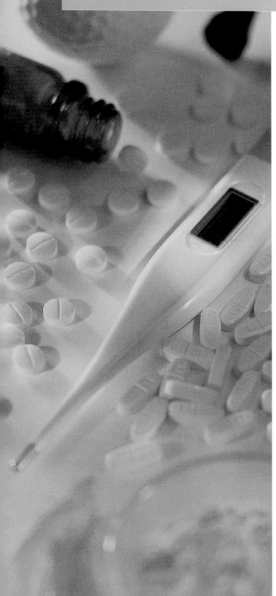

Among the most debilitating conditions, viral infections can be alleviated by a number of complementary therapies, home remedies and dietary regimes. Keeping your immune system in good health can help to prevent viruses from taking hold.

THE PROBLEM

Viruses are microorganisms which cause a wide range of diseases from colds and influenza to AIDS and some forms of cancer. Chickenpox, cold sores, shingles and glandular fever are all viral illnesses.

The virus, which has a core of nucleic acid surrounded by protein, invades weakened cells of the body and multiplies within them, eventually causing their death. When this happens on a large enough scale, large areas of tissue may be severely damaged or even destroyed. Local or general symptoms of inflammation or fever may occur indicating that the body's immune system is at work, as its defensive cells attempt to destroy the invading viruses.

Once the immune system recognises a virus as being harmful it can produce antibodies against future invaders of the same type of virus. However, many viruses can also transform themselves into strains that the immune system cannot recognise, or more virulent strains that may cause more severe health problems.

Most viral illnesses are extremely debilitating, placing great demands on the body's energy reserves. The increased burden of detoxification placed on the liver and organs of elimination may leave feelings of sluggishness and lethargy which are often worsened by the treatments commonly used to relieve infections.

SYMPTOMS

▶ Fever
▶ Inflammation of specific areas of the body
▶ Fatigue, lethargy and constant tiredness
▶ Pain and aching muscles
▶ Swollen glands

IMMUNE HEALTH FACTORS

Certain factors have a detrimental effect on the immune system.

▶ *Alcohol depresses vitamin B and zinc levels which are essential to immune competence. It can also reduce the uptake of several other crucial nutrients.*

▶ *Cigarette smoking actually raises the white blood cell count, activating the immune system. However, smoking also induces low grade chronic bronchitis.*

▶ *Toxic foci – areas of localised infection, such as dental abscesses or infected tonsils – may disturb the normal processes of neutralisation and elimination and weaken the cellular defence.*

▶ *The repeated use of drugs, such as steroids and broad-spectrum antibiotics to treat infections, destroys beneficial acidophilus bacteria in the gut which play an important defensive role.*

▶ *Deficiencies of many nutrients, especially protein, vitamins and minerals, have been associated with depression of the immune system.*

▶ *Prolonged stress reduces the effectiveness of the immune system and is often a contributing factor to a weakened immune response.*

▶ *Excessive exercise may depress the immune system.*

▶ *Lack of natural daylight is associated with a greater level of illness and infection.*

IMMUNE SYSTEM FUNCTIONING

Our bodies have a sophisticated defence system which consists of specialised cells found in the lymph glands, spleen, bone marrow, intestines and lungs. These tissues produce white blood cells which either engulf invading viruses or bacteria or produce antibodies which neutralise foreign cells. The sinuses, lungs and intestines are lined with immunoglobulins and blood levels can be measured to assess immune activity.

We are born with passive immunity, a basic system of defence cells ready to deal with invaders of almost any sort. This non-specific immunity is reinforced through the breast milk. Further immunity is acquired through the formation of antibodies to specific viral attacks, particularly the childhood illnesses, such as measles and chickenpox.

Why do viral illnesses occur?

Many factors can undermine our immunity. In the past, poor standards of hygiene and inadequate nutrition were held responsible for the major epidemics, and to a great extent this is still true of many less developed areas of the world.

Now, however, diseases of excess are more prevalent in the developed world. Excesses of food processing, of chemical residues in food, and even of hygiene in the preoccupation with sterility resulting in the overprescription of antibiotics, have all contributed to the gradual erosion of immune competence. In addition, other aspects of the modern lifestyle, such as heating, air conditioning, electromagnetic radiation and atmospheric pollution, have all been implicated in the growing susceptibility to viral illnesses.

Preventing viral infections

Although there are many factors which increase the susceptibility to infections, and avoiding them will undoubtedly help, there are also a number of measures which sustain and strengthen immune response, such as herbalism and naturopathy.

HERBAL REMEDIES

A herbalist may include herbs to support vulnerable organs as well as those to stimulate immunity.

▶ *Coneflower (*Echinacea angustifolia) *stimulates non-specific resistance. Take a dose of 10–20 drops of tincture dissolved in hot water, three times daily for two to three weeks.*

▶ *Ginseng (*Panax ginseng) *contains adaptogens which help the body to adjust to infections and stress. It is usually available as the crude herb root (steep a slice in hot water daily to use as a tea) or tablets of varying strength (use maximum recommended by the manufacturer).*

▶ *Liquorice (*Glycyrrhiza glabra) *is an adrenal tonic and stimulates the formation of white blood cells and antibodies.*

▶ *Garlic (*Allium sativum) *is an antiseptic and blood cleanser, good for catarrhal infections. For best results, use the tablets prepared from freeze-dried garlic.*

SELF-HELP FOR IMMUNE SUPPORT

There are a number of general measures which you can take to stimulate your resistance to viral infections or to help recovery when they are difficult to shake off. Many are simply common sense, based on the underlying principles of good health – exercise, relaxation and a nutritious diet.

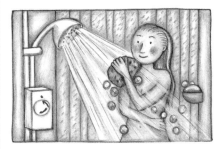

HYDROTHERAPY
Regular cold baths or showers have a protective effect. A study comparing university students who had a daily cold bath with those who did not showed that the cold bath takers had significantly fewer colds.

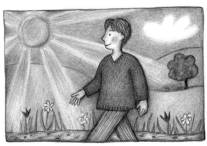

LIGHT
Evidence that people working under artificial light suffer from more infections than those exposed to natural light points to the importance of sunlight to health. It is well known that sunlight is essential for the formation of vitamin D.

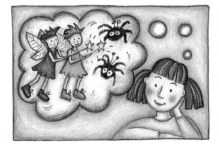

VISUALISATION
Guided imagery is where the patient focuses thoughts on the body's defences using images appropriate to his or her interests. For example, a child might imagine a team of fairies chasing a virus out of the blood.

DIETARY ADVICE

If you are prone to recurrent viral infections the first recommendation is to review your eating habits. Avoid those foods and drinks which are proven suppressors of immunity and have regular meals with plenty of fresh vegetables and fruit, raw whenever possible, and wholegrain produce. Particular foods may need to be increased or reduced for specific types of viral infection, such as herpes, for which foods containing the amino acid arginine (for example nuts and seeds) need to be reduced and those containing the amino acid lysine (for example yoghurt and cottage cheese) need to be increased.

There are also many foods which should feature regularly in your diet for their immune-sustaining and potentiating effects. Garlic and onions have antibacterial and antifungal properties. They also contain sulphur compounds which support detoxification functions of the liver. Live yoghurt contains lactic acid bacteria which have immune supportive properties. Lacto-fermented vegetable juices also provide lactic acid bacteria. Raw vegetables and fruits are rich in antioxidant nutrients such as vitamin C and E, which protect cells against damage and invasion. Brazil nuts provide selenium, an important trace element for immune support and improved functioning. Eat a few nuts several times a week. Also include pumpkin seeds for their zinc and essential fatty acids. A handful with salad or muesli or as a snack is a convenient way of taking them.

One of the most important ways of improving resistance to infections is through dietary modification together with other measures such as hydrotherapy, nutritional supplements and herbal medicines. For the most appropriate way of integrating these for your personal requirements consult a registered naturopath.

SUPPLEMENTS

Keeping your body healthy and working to its best potential is an important aspect of immune protection against viral diseases, and a wide range of vitamins, minerals and trace elements play important roles in immune protection. Care should be taken to avoid an overdose of supplements. Many nutrients may have negative physiological effects if too much is absorbed.

▶ *Vitamin B complex is the most important supplement, which can be taken at 100 mg of a full strength, yeast-free vitamin B.*

▶ *Vitamin C should be taken at a dose of 500 mg of a bioflavonoid complex twice daily.*

▶ *Two 30 mg zinc citrate tablets should be taken at night.*

▶ *Selenium is best taken in the combined formulation with vitamins A, C and E.*

MAKING YOUR OWN JUICES

The raw juices of vegetables and fruits are an excellent source of vitamins, minerals, trace elements and enzymes. They are easy to take and generally very digestible, although the diabetic should be wary (see page 143). Juices are, however, a good way to increase the level of antioxidant nutrients in the diet and may be used as an aperitif or a refreshing between-meal drink. Take a tumblerful at a time and sip the juice slowly. If you have a juicer, freshly pressed juices are best but canned or bottled juices are also good, so long as they are free of any additives or sweeteners (dilute pineapple juice half and half with water).

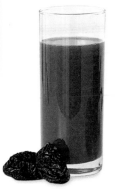

Prune juice provides beta-carotene, potassium and iron, excellent for boosting all-round health and vitality. It is also a useful laxative.

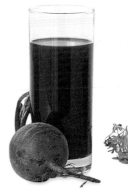

Beetroot juice provides beta-carotene, folic acid, magnesium, potassium, calcium and iron. It may help blood disorders.

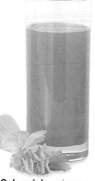

Carrot juice contains folic acid, vitamins A and C, potassium, magnesium and phosphorus. You should limit intake if diabetic.

Celery juice gives you potassium. It is good for lowering high blood pressure and rebalancing adrenal disorders.

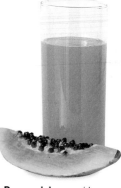

Papaya juice provides vitamin C, beta-carotene, phosphorus and potassium. It is also good for digestion problems.

INDEX

—A—

Abnormal endometrial tissue 35
Acquired immune deficiency
    syndrome 148
Acupressure points 70, 131
Acupuncture 48, 73
Addiction 78
Addison's disease 138
Adrenal cortex 28
Adrenal glands 25, 28, 36
    problems of the 138–9
Adrenaline 21, 25, 107, 138
Aerobic exercise 19, 21, 112
AIDS 148–9
Alcohol 23, 32, 36, 37, 55, 77,
    78, 80
Allergic tension-fatigue
    syndrome 65
Allergies and intolerances 64
Alzheimer's disease 103
Amino acids 107
Anabolic processes 21
Anabolic steroids 80
Anaemia 72, 136–7
Anaerobic exercise 19, 112
Anaphylactic shock 65
Angina pectoris 132
Anorexia nervosa 74
Antibiotic drugs 34, 64
Antidepressant drugs 78, 79
Antidiabetic herbs 143
Antiepileptic drugs 78
Antimalarial drugs 46
Antipsychotic drugs 78
Antithiamin substances 96
Antivomiting drugs 78
Anxiety 60, 62
Aphrodisiac 27, 37
Apnoea 55, 58
Appetite and behaviour 75
Aromatherapy oils 37
Arthritis 47, 70, 71
Ashtanga vinyasa yoga 116–18
Aspirin 78, 79
Asthma 134
Astrology 30, 49, 52
    Chinese 52
    Western 49
Autoimmune disorder 69
Ayurveda 48, 50–51
Ayurvedic treatments 48

—B—

Bach flower remedies 46
Back pain 69
Basal metabolic rate (BMR) 21
Beetroot juice 156
Behavioural changes 29, 122
Benign prostatic hypertrophy 38

Biodynamic theory 25
Birthing positions 31
Blood cell formation 95
Blood circulation 113
Blood pressure 130–1
Bowen technique 68
Brain function 43
Breakfast 88
Breathing exercise 113
Breathing problems 71
Bronchitis 134
Bulimia 74
Burnout 63
Butterflies and navigation 43

—C—

Caffeine 23, 32, 73, 77, 80,
    86
Calcium 31, 85
Calorie-controlled diet 21
Calories 82, 85
Cancer 42, 146–7
Candida or thrush 34
Cardiovascular strength
    95
Carnitine 105
Catabolism 21
Cataplexy 56
Cauliflower 5, 104
Celery juice 156
Chanting to relieve
    depression 45
Chi kung 48, 120, 123
Chinese astrology 49, 52
Chiropractic 69, 71
Chlorosis 74
Choline 103
Chromium deficiency
    and diabetes 92
Chronic fatigue 62, 72
Chronic fatigue immune
    deficiency syndrome
    (CFIDS) 150
Chronic fatigue syndrome
    (CFS) 150
Chronic pain 68
Clinical depression 60
Codeine 78, 80
Coenzyme Q10 86, 109, 139,
    153
    and ageing 109
Colds 51
Colour therapy 42
Complex carbohydrates 20, 83,
    86, 87
Computed tomography 42
Computer screens 67
Constipation 26, 71
Contraceptive pill 34, 79
Copper bracelets for arthritis 47

Coronary artery 132
Corticosteroid hormones 138
Cortisol 25, 28
Cough medicines 80, 135
Counselling 35, 51, 126
Crash diets 74
Crystals 47
Crystal therapy 47
Cystitis 34

—D—

Dairy products 19
Daytime drowsiness 55, 76
Daytime performance 54
Dental devices 59
Depression 26, 45, 60, 99, 100
Diabetes 28, 92, 142–3
    dietary measures for 143
Diarrhoea 26, 71, 72
Diastolic pressure 130
Dietary advice 77, 82
Dieting and weight control 72
Diets that drain energy 72
Digestion 18
    enzymes 83
    juices 18
    timescale 18
Disaccharides 19
DNA 102
Dopamine 78, 107
Dreaming period 54
Dreams 56
Drowsiness 76
Drugs 36, 60, 78
    and emotions 60
    and food interactions 79
    and workability 80
    that drain energy 78

—E—

Earth's magnetic field 43
Eastern exercise traditions 117
Ejaculation 38
Elderly people 21
Electrical charge 42
Electro-crystal therapy 47
Electromagnetic
    field therapy (EMF) 43
    radiation 40
    spectrum 40
    wavelength 40
Electromagnetism 43
Emotional
    drain on energy 60
    effects of colour 41
    factors 75
    phases 32
    problems 60
    stress 113

Emotions 113, 119
    and energy 60, 119
Emphysema 134
Endocrine system 24, 26, 28
Endocrinologist 26
Endocrinology courses 26
Endometriosis 35
Endorphins 25, 64
Energy
    and activity 19
    and animals 46
    and cultural factors 28, 44
    and nature 38
    and your body 18
    and your emotions 60, 119
    draining 122
    laws of 16
    levels and drinks 77
    levels and special diets 90
    levels through the day 88
    needs for men 36
    needs for women 22
    nutrients 94
    production 95
    requirements 20
        and age 22
    transfer 19
Enlarged prostate 38
Environmental factors 17, 24,
    66, 67
Enzymes 18
Epstein-Barr virus (EBV) 150
Evening primrose oil 86
Exercise 17, 19, 23, 32, 55,
    112, 151
    aerobic 19, 21, 112
    anaerobic 19, 112
Exhaustion 122

—F—

Fatigue 62, 72
    avoiding during day 76
Fats 19, 82, 84
    saturated 82, 84
    unsaturated 82, 84
Fat-soluble vitamins 94
Fatty acids 20, 84
Female
    energy needs 22
    hormones 29
    reproductive system 29
Feng shui 66
Fish oils 70
Five element theory 49
Five elements and Chinese
    astrology 52
Five principal forces of
    energy 48
Flower remedies 46
Fluorine 85

Folic acid 31, 85, 86, 101, 102, 136
Food
  allergies 69
  cravings 34
  intolerances 64
  supplements 133
Friendship 126
Fruit and vegetables 82

—G—

Gall bladder 18
Gamma linolenic acid 30
Gamma rays 40
Garlic 86
Genetic
  factors 28, 67
  makeup 67
Gingko biloba 86
Ginseng 86, 139
Glands 22, 24
Glandular fever 153
Glandular problems 138
Glucose 18, 20, 21, 32, 83
Glycerol 20
Glyceryl trinitrate (GTN) 133
Glycogen 20
Goitre 140
Grass pollen 64
Grief 60
Growth hormone 25
Growth spurt 24

—H—

Haemoglobin 136
Half-fat milk 75
Hallucinations 56
Happiness 30
Hayfever 64
Headaches 71
Headaches and sinus
  problems 51
Health and happiness 35
Heart 112, 132–3
  and artery disease 132–3
  attack 132, 133
  disease 132
Heat 40
Herbal
  medicine 139
  remedies 51, 155
Herbalism 48
High blood pressure 130–1
High-intensity lasers 42
HIV and AIDS 148–9
Homeopathy 46, 139, 141, 153
Hormonal
  changes 28, 29, 33, 55, 88
  complications 27
  glands 24
  replacement therapy 28, 34
Hormone regulation 25
Hormones 25, 26, 83

House dust mite 65
Human immunodeficiency
  virus (HIV) 148–9
Humidity 67
Hydrotherapy 131, 155
Hypersensitivity 64
Hypersomnia 55
Hypertension 130
Hyperthyroidism 140
Hypoglycaemia 84, 138, 144–5
Hypotension 130
Hypothalamus 24, 25, 28, 62
Hypothalamus-pituitary
  system 27, 62
Hypothyroidism 140

—I—

Ibuprofen 78, 80
Imaging technique 44
Immune system 64, 155
Impotence 37
Increased urinary output 26
Indigestion 51, 71
Infection tests 128
Infertility 34
Infrared waves 40
Insomnia 55
Insulin 21, 84, 142, 144
Insulin-dependent diabetes
  (IDD) 92, 142
Intolerances 64
Iodine 85
Iron 31, 85, 86, 106, 137
  deficiency 72, 137
Irritability 29, 30

—J—

Jet lag 56
Jin Shin 71
Juices
  beetroot 156
  celery 156
  papaya 156
  prune 156

—K—

Keeping fit 31
Kilocalories 18, 19, 82, 88, 92
Kinetic energy 16
Krebs cycle 84

—L—

Large intestine 18, 34
Laudanum 78
Laws of energy 16
Leg joints 68
Libido 37
Lifestyle 20, 35, 58
Light 40, 67, 155
  and colour 17, 40

in medicine 40
  therapy 40
Lightning 17, 42
Losing weight 93
Love 29
Low blood pressure 130–1
Low-intensity lasers 42
Low testosterone levels 36
Lung disorders 134–5
Lymphatic system 113

—M—

Macronutrients in vegetarian
  diets 90
Magnesium 30, 72, 85, 86, 110, 139, 153
  supplements 94
Magnetic
  force 43
  navigation 43
  resonance imaging (MRI) 43
  rocks 43
Magnetising water 43
Magnetism 43
Magnet therapy 43
Malaria 46
Male
  energy needs 22, 36
  growth spurt 24
  reproductive system 36
Manipulative therapies 69, 71
Massage
  and aromatherapy oils 37
  therapies 48, 69, 70, 71
ME (myalgic encephalomyelitis)
  150–3
Medical tests 128
Medication 78
Meditation 51
  standing 121, 123
Mediterranean diet 74
Melanin 107
Melatonin 25
Men and energy 36
Menopause 27, 34
  and energy levels 27
Menstruation 25, 29, 30, 68, 136
Mental attitude 49, 112
Mental relaxation 62
Metabolic changes 29
Metabolism 19, 21, 28, 29, 31, 33, 43, 74, 83
Metal 48, 49
Migraines 68
Mind–body link 118
Minerals 46, 47, 83, 85, 94
Mitochondria 105
Monosaccharide 19
Monounsaturated fats 84
Mood swings 30
Morning sickness 32
Morphine 78
Muscle

activity 43
  damage 71
  pain 71
Music and song 44

—N—

Naproxen 78
Narcolepsy 55
Negativism 30
Nervous system functioning 95
Neurochemicals 89
Neurons 60
Neuropeptides 118
Neurotransmitters 68, 78, 103, 107
Niacin 31, 85, 98
Nicotine 32, 80
Nicotinic acid 98
Noise 67
Non-insulin dependent diabetes 142
Noradrenaline 25, 107, 138
Nursing mothers 20

—O—

Obesity 20, 28, 74
Oestrogen 25, 29, 98
Oily fish 98
Opium 78, 80
Osteoarthritis 68
Osteopathy 69, 71
Ovarian dysfunction 34
Ovaries 24, 25, 33, 94
Over-the-counter drugs 79
Overweight 19, 28, 37, 74

—P—

Pain 69
  diary 69
  in the joints 68
  receptors 69
  transmission 69
Painkillers 78, 80
Pancreas 18, 24, 25
Pantothenic acid 99
Papaya juice 156
Paracetamol 79
Passive smoking 66
Pellagra 98
Penicillin 64
Period pains 71, 80
Phosphorus 31
Phosphorylcreatine 19
Physiotherapy 44, 69, 71
Phytates 106
Pickwickian Syndrome 55
Pineal gland 25
Pituitary gland 24, 25, 28
Pneumoconiosis 134
Pollen 64
  grass 64
  levels through the day 64

plant 64
tree 64
weed 64
Polyunsaturated fats 84
Polysaccharides 19
Potassium 85
Pregnancy 20, 28, 29, 30, 31, 32, 55
Premenstrual fatigue 30
Premenstrual syndrome (PMS) 29, 100
Prescription drugs 78
Progesterone 25, 29
Progesterone-only pill 79
Prostate gland 36
problems 27, 38
Proteins 19, 22, 31, 82, 85
Prune juice 156
Psychiatric disorders 60
Psychological conditions 27
Puberty 36
Pyridoxine (see vitamin B$_6$) 100

—Q—

Quartz crystals 47
Quinine 46

—R—

Radiation therapy 17
Radiotherapy 40, 42
Radiowaves 40
Rational emotive therapy 61
Recipes
Baked trout with lemon 98
Bruschetta with cold roast beef 106
Calf's liver and bacon 101
Chicken liver pâté with wholemeal toast 97
Eggs benedict 107
Fruit salad 104
Grilled chicken and pepper rosetti 100
Kebabs with grilled vegetables 105
Mixed leaf salad with cheese and wholegrain roll 103
Moules mariniere 108
Sardine and olive pasta bake 109
Spicy chicken tortillas 99
Tofu with chinese vegetables 96
Tuscan bean soup 102
Recreational drugs 80
Red wine 74
Reiki 71
Reincarnation 50
Relationships 17
Relaxation 37
benefits of 37
techniques 55, 61

REM sleep 54
Reproduction 24
female system 29
male system 36
Restricted diets 99
Rheumatic pain 71
Rheumatism 47
Rheumatoid arthritis 69, 80
Riboflavin 31, 85, 91, 97
Rose quartz 47

—S—

St John's wort 71
Saturated fat 82, 84
Scanning and positron emission tomography 42
Schizophrenia 100
Scurvy and vitamin C deficiency 104
Seasonal affective disorder (SAD) 40, 48, 67
Seaweed 120
Selenium 86, 153
Semiprecious stones 47
Serotonin levels 107
Sex 17, 117
Sexual behaviour 50
Shiatsu 71
Shiftwork 57
Siestas 55
Silver 47
Singing 44, 151
Skin cancer 42
Skin changes 29
Sleep 23, 54
and alcohol 57
and apnoea 55, 58
and snoring 55, 58
deep 56
Small intestine 18
Smoking 37, 80
Smoky quartz 47
Snoring 55, 58
and apnoea 55, 58
devices that help 58
Sodium 85
Somnambulism 56
Sound 44
therapy 44, 45
Space-clearing 62
Special diets 90
Spiritual health 50, 62, 102
Spring cleaning 62
Standing meditation 121, 123
Steroids 21, 34, 80
Stomach ulcers 71
Stress 35, 62, 122
management 141
Stretching 76, 116
Sugars 82
Sunstroke 42
Supplements 30, 86
Support mechanisms 126

—T—

Teenagers and energy levels 21
Teeth and bones 46
Temperature factors 66
Testicular atrophy 36
Testosterone 25, 28, 36, 80
replacement 36
Thai massage 71
Thiamin 31, 72, 85, 96
Throat problems 71
Thrush infection 34
Thymus 24
Thyroid glands 25, 140–1
disease 28
disorders 27
factors 140–1
hormones 107
and parathyroids 24
problems 140–1
stimulating hormone (TSI I) 140
test 128
Thyroxin (T4) 21, 25, 140
Tibetan Buddhism 121
Touch therapies 70
Traditional Chinese medicine 46, 48, 75, 90
Travel sickness pills 78
Tryptophan 89, 98, 107
Tui Na 48, 70
TV screens 67
Tyrosine 107

—U—

Ultrasonic sounds 47
Ultrasound 44
Ultraviolet light 40
Unsaturated fats 82, 84
Urine test 128

—V—

Vegan diet 74, 90
Vegetable oils 19
Vegetarian diets 74, 90, 91
and nutrients 91
lacto 90
lacto-ovo 90
Viral infections 154–6
Visualisation 155
Vital force 46
Vitamin
A 31, 86, 135
B complex 86, 99, 103, 137, 139, 145, 153, 156
B$_1$ see Thiamin
B$_2$ see Riboflavin
B$_3$ see Niacin
B$_5$ see Pantothenic acid
B$_6$ 30, 31, 38, 97, 100
B$_{12}$ 72, 91, 101, 136
C 31, 86, 104, 105, 135, 136, 137, 139, 153, 156

C deficiency and scurvy 104
D 31, 91
E 31, 86, 153
Vitamins 31, 85, 94, 95
and minerals for pregnancy 31
fat-soluble 94
water-soluble 94

—W—

Water-soluble vitamins 94
Weather 66
Weight change 26, 29
Weight watching 17
Wine 74
Women and energy 29

—X—

X-rays 40, 42
and radiation 42

—Y—

Yin and yang 49
foods 75
Ylang ylang essential oil 37
Yoga 51, 55, 116
Yoghurt 34, 77

—Z—

Zinc 27, 38, 72, 86, 108, 135, 153
and the immune system 108
and libido 27

ACKNOWLEDGMENTS

Carroll & Brown Limited
would like to thank
Rachel Aris
Dr Edward Bach Centre
Bowtech
International Association for Colour
  Therapy
Michael Tse, Tse Qigong Centre

Photographic assistants
Lee McPherson
Colin Tatham
M.A. Hugo

Picture research
Richard Soar

Index
Jennifer Mussett

Photograph sources
6 The Stock Market
9 (Top) Science Photo Library
  (Bottom) US Library of
  Congress/Science Photo Library
10 Oriental Museum, Durham
  University, UK/Bridgeman Art
  Library, London
11 Science Photo Library
12 Tony Stone Images
21 Tony Stone Images
26 (Top) Chris Priesti/Science
  Photo Library
  (Bottom) Wellcome Institute
  Library, London
28 Hutchison Library
34 (Left) E. Gueho/CNRI Science
  Photo Library
  (Right) Professor P.M. Motta
  et al/Science Photo Library
36 The Image Bank
40 The Image Bank
43 (Left) Scott Camazine/Science
  Photo Library
  (Centre) The Stock Market
  (Top right) Sinclair Stammers/
  Science Photo Library
  (Right) Professor P.M. Motta
  et al/Science Photo Library
  (Bottom right) Claude
  Nuridsany & Marie Perennou/
  Science Photo Library
44 (Top) Charron, Jerrican/Science
  Photo Library
  (Bottom) Corbis/Hulton
  Deutsche Collection
45 Tibet Images
46 Dr Edward Bach Centre
46 The Image Bank
48 Pictor International
49 (Wood) Pictor International
  (Metal) Pictor International
50 Science Museum/Science &
  Society Picture Library
54 Kunsthistorisches Museum,
  Vienna/Bridgeman Art Library,
  London
55 Tony Stone Images
57 Tony Stone Images
62 The Stock Market
63 Tony Stone Images
65 Eye of Science/Science Photo
  Library
67 Elizabeth Whiting Associates/
  Andrew Kolesnikow
68 Bowtech
74 (Top) Smith Art Gallery and
  Museum, Stirling/Bridgeman Art
  Library, London
  (Bottom) Tony Stone Images
76 Tony Stone Images
78 Tony Stone Images
95 (Left) Andrew Syred/Science
  Photo Library
  (Right) CNRI/Science Photo
  Library
112 The Stock Market
123 Michael Tse, Tse Qigong Centre
126 Tony Stone Images
128 The Stock Market
132 The Stock Market
136 Dr Gopal Murti/Science Photo
  Library
149 NIBSC/Science Photo Library

Illustrators
Kim Dalziel
Rosamund Fowler
John Geary
Nicola Gregory
Halli Verinder
Anthea Whitworth
Paul Williams

Hair and make-up
Bettina Graham
Kim Menzies

075–015–01